A Tear from My Heart

Note: The personal experiences shared in this book are not intended to be used in the diagnosis or treatment of any disease. Please consult your physician with medical questions and concerns.

© Copyright Carlisle Press March 2008

ISBN 10-digit: 1-933753-06-4
ISBN 13-digit: 978-1-933753-06-5

Book and Cover Design: Amy Wengerd
Book Printing: Carlisle Printing

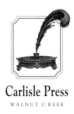

Carlisle Press
WALNUT CREEK

2701 TR 421
Sugarcreek, OH 44681

Acknowledgments

A HEARTY THANK-YOU to all the women who were willing to share a part of their lives. Without your help this book would not have been possible. I believe many emotions were stirred and tears shed over the writing and reliving of these traumatic experiences. It is our hope and prayer that this book may be an inspiring and encouraging book to all who have had this experience. We also hope that through these stories others may be warned of the symptoms of ectopics.

A thank-you to the authors of the poems in this book. May they also be a help in comforting hurting women.

Above all, we thank God for sparing our lives, for allowing us the privilege to tell our stories. If they can be even a small comfort to grieving mothers, give God the glory!

Table of Contents

To Encourage You

Beloved friend, my heart is pained
To think of what you're facing.
I'm sure you wonder why this is,
What plan our God is tracing.
You wonder what the future holds,
And if your heart can bear
The burdens and the suffering
That seem your constant share.

You wonder what He'd have you learn
And where you need correction;
Your way seems dark, you cannot see
Which is the right direction.
Your days are long, your nights are dark,
Your mind is worn from thinking,
Sometimes it seems as if your faith
Were vanishing and sinking.

Lift up your eyes and praise His name
And meet the Lord in prayer.
This is God's will; He knows it all,
And you are in His care.
He sees you as a precious gem
That with some slight correction,
Some polishing and grinding, too,
Can almost reach perfection.

He wants to burn the dross away,
To prune unfruitful vine,
To mold you as the potter's clay
Into a vessel fine.
Do not despair! Look up! Fight on!
The way will someday show;
And later on, when life is past,
You will the reason know.

The Lord would test and strengthen you,
And fit you for His task;
You cannot serve Him fully while
In easy life you bask.
You know not what tomorrow holds,
You know who holds tomorrow,
So live in faith, just for today,
Though it is filled with sorrow.

God loves you still; He holds your hand;
Just cling to Him secure
And fully, sweetly trust Him and
This, too, you shall endure!
—*Mrs. Silas Bowman*

Dreams Laid Away

We thought the days ahead would bring
Once more to us the wondrous joy
Of tiny, dimpled baby hands,
Belonging to a little boy,
Or little girl. We did not know—
We did not care; it mattered not.
Whichever God would choose to send
Would add a blessing to our lot.

We thought the days ahead would bring
More love, almost, than hearts could hold.
We dreamed of tiny sleepers, warm,
And blankets, shielding from the cold.
Our minds had pictured sharp and clear
(As if it were reality!)
The first time that our eyes would meet
And we a precious smile would see.

We dreamed of all the countless things
Our other children, dear, would say;
Of all the eager helping hands
That would be close, throughout the day;
Of how they'd watch the clock to see
Whose turn was next, in rocking chair,
To hold that tiny bundle, sweet,
And gently touch the silky hair.

All this we dreamed—and yet...and yet...
God had another plan in mind.
His ways are not our ways, and so
We leave our precious dreams behind.
We gently lay them all aside—
(They were so very real, so dear!)
Dreams are but shadows of the best...
God's best for us is now made clear.

We want that best, our Father God,
So in Thy hands we place it all.
Our love seems great—but Thine is more!
Our dreams are only foretastes small
Of all the wonders Thou hast planned,
For us, and for our lives while here.
We need not always understand.
Someday, Thou wilt make all things clear!
—*L.B*

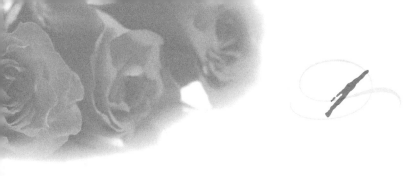

Flowers for the Master's Bouquet

—anonymous, Dundee, NY

"GUESS WHAT? I'M pregnant!" I happily announced to my husband. Even though I had not done a pregnancy test yet, I felt sure my suspicions were correct, as I had skipped a period and was experiencing all the usual symptoms. We eagerly counted the months until this new miracle, Lord willing, would be added to our family of two boys. How exciting it would be for all of us!

Several days later, while shopping, I purchased several pregnancy kits, just to make sure I really was pregnant before we shared the news with our families.

Once at home again, I did one of the tests, confident that we would get a positive result. But wait—something was not right—it showed negative! "Must be I drank too much water," I guessed to my husband. Later in the day, he begged me to try the other test. Surely this time it would show positive. But once again we were greatly disappointed and puzzled with a negative result.

"Really, can you depend on the accuracy of these cheap tests? Why don't we try a good-quality test from the pharmacy before we give up?" I asked. So that very same week we bought two more at the pharmacy. Tensely, we waited for the pink plus sign which we knew would appear. But for the third time we were disappointed.

The next day was a repeat. Whatever could be wrong? Surely these symptoms I'd been experiencing were not just my imagination. We read all the instructions on the sheet, searching for any clues to our puzzle. "An ectopic pregnancy can cause a false or irregular result with your test," we read. Was this the problem?

Several months before, I had heard of one lady's life-threatening experience with ectopics. Remembering this, my husband urged, "Let's go for an ultrasound tomorrow. I don't want you to pass out while I'm at work."

But first we wanted to get a second opinion, because, after all, ultrasounds were expensive. So I asked my mom for advice. She calmed our fears by assuring us that if I had no pain, there should be nothing to worry about, as the pain of ectopics is worse than childbirth. Since I was feeling as fine as ever, we dropped the thought of a tubal pregnancy.

And then it happened—I had a period two weeks late. A late period was nothing new to me, since before our marriage they had ranged anywhere from 3-13 weeks, although they had been very regular after our marriage. Thus we determined that all the symptoms were just imaginary and we totally dismissed the thoughts of my being pregnant. How could I be pregnant if I was still getting my period? It seemed like a very normal one.

(Later we were told that with an ectopic, there are not enough hormones to signal the body to quit menstruating.)

Ten days later I had light spotting and slight pressure for three days. Since I wasn't pregnant, it didn't scare me, and I passed it off as a light, abnormal period.

For a whole week afterward I was fine, but then, on a Thursday, I was invited to a neighborhood quilting. I chose to stay at home, as our 18-month-old was croupy. Shortly after lunch, I felt a fierce pressure in my rectal area. Lying on the sofa, I tried in vain to ease the severe pain. Sitting was out of the question with the searing, burning pain. How thankful I was that I was in my own home instead of with a room full of ladies, wondering what ails me!

During this time, our youngest son begged and begged to nurse, but the poor little boy—all I could do was push him away from my painful abdomen. After about an hour, though, the pain gradually left, and soon I felt able to tuck the boys into their beds, tackle the dishes and continue with the day's work.

For the following two days I felt fine, but of course we tried to figure out what may have caused the pain. We thought it may have been something I was eating, so I changed my diet to all fruits and vegetables.

On Sunday we stayed home from church, as by that time, our oldest son (age 3) was running a fever of 103°. Again, I was extremely thankful to be in the comfort of our own home, as that morning, I had another painful attack, accompanied by another hour of lying on the sofa, trying to cope with the pain.

After the pain had subsided somewhat, I felt weak, but I got up anyway. "You look as if you could use some fresh air," my husband told me. "Would you like to fill the outdoor furnace?"

"Sure," I agreed, glad for a chance to get outside. But, walking out to the furnace, I wasn't so sure after all. With the ever-present dull ache in my abdomen, I had to walk slowly and carefully, and I couldn't even stand up straight. Picking up pieces of firewood was indeed a chore—each piece seemed to weigh tons. But I did get the task done, and eventually the pain subsided even more. (If my husband would have known what a chore this would be for me, he would never even have suggested it!) It was during this bout of pain that I began spotting again.

On Monday I was back to "normal" again, but on Tuesday having done my morning work, and with the two boys sitting where they could watch me, I began sewing at a quilt I was piecing.

However, after only fifteen minutes of sewing, intense pain raged through my body again. It felt as if someone were turning a knife in my insides. Moaning, I stumbled to my usual haunt of the past few days—the sofa. I lay there all forenoon, with my poor little boy begging to nurse, and both boys bumping around me. What ailed their mom anyway, neglecting them and pushing them away?

By sheer determination and gritting of teeth, I somehow managed to warm up something for dinner (while bent over with pain), feed the boys and put them to bed for their naps. It was all I could do to pick up our youngest son and deposit him into his crib.

I flopped across our bed and wept my heart out. The stress of all this pain and wondering what was wrong with me was getting the best of me. Was it stress that was causing the pain? I knew stress could react in strange ways. Or was it appendicitis? My sister had it only a year before, which is why the idea came to my mind.

I called her and we compared the way our pains acted. In a way, it sounded almost same, and yet, it seemed different. It couldn't be a tubal pregnancy, as I'd just had a period several weeks before. I really wasn't ready to call a doctor, as the pain would probably leave for good soon, and I'd be back to normal.

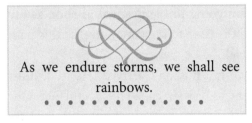

As we endure storms, we shall see rainbows.

· · · · · · · · · · · · · ·

Finally, around 3:00 I felt able to tackle the dishes. While I was slowly getting the kitchen back in order, the boys were happily playing with some kitchen utensils on the floor. When I had my back turned, they pulled out all three drawers in the cabinet beside the stove, causing the cabinet to fall forward on top of their legs.

Shaking and feeling weak, I set the cabinet back into place and was checking to see if our screaming boys were all right, when my dear husband walked in the door. What a fright met his eyes! His wife, white as a sheet, was trying to comfort two screaming boys. Needless to say, the cabinet was securely fastened within minutes!

The next day, Wednesday, I was invited to a neighborhood comfort knotting. With the boys just getting over the flu and not knowing when I would get another "attack," we again stayed at home.

I felt fine until around 11:30, when we'd just started eating dinner. Fierce pain shot through my body, worse than ever before. (And, I decided later, definitely worse than childbirth.) I clutched my stomach and moaned and groaned as I slumped in my chair. Our oldest son sat on his stool, imitating me. Did he think I was playing a game?!

I dragged myself to the sofa, trying in vain to ease the pain by pushing a pillow against my right side, where the pain was worse. I never even thought of getting help; I was so preoccupied with coping with the pain. This time I became feverish, sweating one minute and shivering the next.

How I hoped and prayed that my dear husband would come home early, as it was during this bout of pain that I made up my mind. "*Today* I am going to the hospital as soon as my husband gets home. It is time to *do* something, as this pain will not go away by itself."

At 3:30, thank God, my husband arrived! He, too, must have decided it's urgent, as he soon called the ambulance. Our next-door neighbor came to stay with the boys until my sister arrived. She was already on her way over.

"Are you pregnant?" the lady on the ambulance asked.

"I very much doubt it. Likely I have appendicitis," I answered.

Once at the hospital, we answered countless questions. A urine test was performed. "The test indicates that you are pregnant," a nurse announced. Needless to say, we were shocked. We just didn't think it was possible.

The nurse had a hard time getting into my vein to hook up IV. She made a remark about my small veins, but no wonder, the amount of blood I'd lost, as we were to discover later. I was given a painkiller and soon felt much better.

Several hours later I was wheeled into a dark room for an ultrasound. The technician was a grumpy male of few words. When my husband asked him a question, he answered with a curt, "Don't talk!"

How we wanted to know what he was finding, for after all, this was *my* body and *my* baby. Eventually he did inform us that the uterus is empty, but there's a mass on my right tube. He arranged to send us to another hospital, twelve miles away, where they were better equipped for such things.

Around 9:00 p.m. we arrived at that hospital, where we faced more questions and paperwork. The doctor scheduled surgery for the following forenoon. He guessed the problem could be one of three things, one of which was an ectopic, but that could not be determined until during surgery. We knew there was not much hope for this baby, as by now we were convinced it must be an ectopic.

At long last I was allowed to crawl into a nice, soft bed, and my husband was given a folding cot. I was so grateful for his comforting presence in these strange surroundings. (I had never before needed to go to the hospital.) It was 12:30 by the time the nurses quit running back and forth to my roommate, and only then could we rest.

Thursday morning, March 23, dawned, after a few fitful hours of sleep in unfamiliar beds. I was given two units of blood before I could go for surgery. This brought the color back to my ashen face! I was just about to be wheeled into the operating room, when both of our moms arrived. They were a welcome sight, especially for my husband, who would have had a long, lonely wait while I was in surgery. He could not keep back the tears of relief and gladness. The past 18 hours had been very stressful for him.

After the nurses heaped a mountain of toasty warm blankets on top of me (I was shivering all over), I was wheeled into a frigidly cold operating room. The next thing I knew, I was reluctantly waking out of a deep sleep. Oh, my stomach was sore! I wished I could go back to sleep and never wake up again! I did not feel ready to face reality.

The doctor guessed my tube had been burst for two weeks already, but my own guess would be one week, as it was only a week since the first horrible pain. My body was one bloody mess, from internal bleeding. My right tube was removed, but the clotted blood was left inside my body, so that I could reabsorb the iron. I was nine weeks along.

I was so groggy when I awoke that my mind could not fully grasp all the doctor told me. When a friend asked, a few days later, if my tube had burst, I honestly did not even know, but I didn't think it had! I had to ask my mom for this bit of information.

By 7:00 that evening, we were safely at home. We were happy to see our boys after being separated for over 24 hours, but with my sister there, they were in good hands and with one whom they knew well.

Because of my three sore half-inch incisions, we decided this would be a good time to wean our youngest. He had only been nursing to go to sleep, so it wasn't a big adjustment for him. It was much harder for me. I regretted our decision, as I began thinking that if he were my last baby, I would nurse him for a good long while yet.

At first we thought we would not grieve for a baby we did not even know we had, until after its tiny soul had entered eternity. But once reality set in, we did grieve, both for our baby and the tube. Like a friend told us, a tubal pregnancy is a double loss. Not only do you lose one you never met, you also give up a tube. We found this to be very true.

My nights were terrible those first months after my surgery. While my tired mind and body should have been resting, my thoughts were spinning like a vicious whirlwind, reliving the events of the tubal pregnancy. Sometimes I so desperately wanted to sleep that I felt like I was losing my mind.

To think how life-threatening an ectopic is, and how long we pushed off doing something, is mind-boggling. I'd wonder about future pregnancies. Would the next one end up in the same dreadful way? Would we ever again have the joy of holding our own newborn baby? Could we ever give our boys the gift of a baby brother or sister? Often it was past midnight until my weary body dropped off to sleep, only to awaken several more times in the wee hours of the morning to lie awake again. It took me *months* to learn to sleep really well.

We appreciated all the mail we received, the meals that were brought in and friends who asked about our experience. I recovered quickly and was soon able to handle the work by myself. But I had a long way to go yet emotionally. That part of the healing process would take much longer.

Sometimes we wondered if God was punishing us. But, no, we decided He had a reason for allowing this to happen and someday we would understand. This was all a part of His divine plan for our lives. Through this ordeal, our first great trial of our married life, we learned to know each other better, as we each grieved in our own way. We came to more fully appreciate our precious boys, for truly children are a miracle we too often take for granted.

In the seven months following my surgery, three sisters-in-law were blessed with babies, two of them being quite close to what would have been my due date. How utterly forsaken and left out I felt. It just did not seem fair that our baby was taken while others were allowed to keep and enjoy theirs. But we knew God was in control and He knew what was best.

"Choose my path, O blessed Saviour,
Let me, trusting, lean on Thee;
Order Thou my steps, dear Saviour,
Just as seemeth good to Thee..."

It was also difficult for me to go to church and see all the expecting mothers and newborn babies. Many Sundays I would cry inwardly, especially when I was extra tired and everything appeared dark and hopeless. I was able to cope much better if I was well rested.

One day in church, only a few weeks after our loss, a friend happily asked if I'd heard her news. With our grief still so fresh and raw, this cut to the core of my being. I wished I could run away and hide. Instead, in an attempt to be happy for them, I asked when it's due.

"We're keeping that a secret," was her reply. What a slap

in the face! I felt crushed. "If I had such wonderful news, I would feel like shouting it to the whole world," I confided to my husband later.

Didn't she realize I was hurting and needed to be "handled carefully"? Of course she didn't—she had no experience in giving up babies. I had to think, "Forgive them, for they know not what they do." It was up to me to forgive her, for after all, the Bible says, "Rejoice with them that do rejoice, and weep with them that weep." Hadn't she sympathized with us when we gave up our dear baby? Many pleas were sent Heavenward as I struggled to overcome wrong feelings.

Amidst the pregnancies and newborns of our family and friends, I found comfort in the thought that our family was now started in Heaven. Oh, if we could only remain faithful till the end and greet our dear one (was it a boy or a girl?) in Heaven some sweet day.

I purchased and read the book *I'll Hold You in Heaven*, and we knew without a doubt that this tiny soul was indeed in Heaven. I'd envision entering those pearly gates and our child would come running to greet us, and we would know him/ her, even though we'd never met.

Another lovely thought was one shared by my aunt who'd encountered numerous miscarriages. She likes to think of these tiny souls as butterflies in Heaven. I loved to envision our own precious butterfly, flitting amongst the glorious flowers in Heaven, in tune with the sweet songs of the angels. Why would we wish our dear one back into this evil, sin-filled world? And yet, our arms ached to hold our baby.

"Some sweet day when life is o'er,
We shall meet above,
We shall greet those gone before,
In that home of love.

Some sweet day, some sweet day,
Oh, that happy time will be,
Some sweet day."

This song was sung at my husband's grandfather's funeral, only seven weeks after my surgery. It was so touching to me.

Every evening our oldest son would ask God to give us a baby. He begged over and over to go to Heaven and get a baby from Jesus for us. How they both loved babies!

After my ectopic, I had the feeling that our trials were not yet over, that God was not yet done refining us. I felt we would have another loss, but in what way, I did not know.

I often longed for the "carefree" days I had before the tubal. My cycle became wacky after the surgery, and whenever my period was late, I'd begin testing right away. When the test showed negative, we feared I was having another tubal. Even after I'd have my period, I'd wonder if everything was actually okay. Sometimes we'd even get a blood test done, just for peace of mind.

We really wanted another baby, yet at the same time, we shrank from the idea. Could we face another loss, if that's how it turned out? Still, we tried, waited, trusted, prayed, hoped...

Six months after my ectopic, my cycle was late again, but I blamed it on the stressful week I'd just had. But just to make sure, I did two tests that week, and like always, they showed negative. The following week I did only

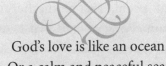

God's love is like an ocean
Or a calm and peaceful sea,
His love dates from creation
It envelops you and me.
We can never overtake it,
We can never use it up,
It is boundless, it is endless,
And it overflows our cup.

one test, for what was the use of wasting so many tests? This one, too, showed negative.

The third week, I did a fourth test, simply because I had one left. This one, as we expected, was also negative. I looked again, and was shocked to see it had changed to a plus sign! We were sure it was a false positive, as I'd had absolutely no symptoms (besides a missed period), but our midwife assured us there's never a false positive.

She did a blood test that very same day to check my HCG levels, which were up to 723, a fairly normal range for six weeks. Two days later we'd do a second test and by then the levels should be doubled, and if not... I didn't even want to think about it.

Could we handle another loss so soon? We did not allow ourselves to get excited about this pregnancy, for we knew there was very little hope, if it took so long to get a positive result. Still, we vaguely hoped for a new little one in our hearts and home.

Two days later, we were crushed when we heard the disappointing results of the second blood test. The HCG level had risen only 25 points to 748. My midwife assured me I may be going to miscarry, since the levels didn't rise more, but it could also be another tubal. When she hung up, I was soon crying so hard that I could barely tell my husband the sad news.

Since this was Friday we'd need to wait for an ultrasound until Monday. The long weekend loomed before us like a dark, forboding cloud. If this was a tubal, and I was almost seven weeks along, my tube could burst at any time...

That night we slept very poorly. The next day we planted a young oak tree in a spot visible from the kitchen window. This tree was in memory of the baby we'd lost in the spring. Our due date, October 23, was just a few days away. Tears were close to the surface as we thought of what could have been.

We managed to feel pretty optimistic throughout the long weekend. I feel it was the prayers of many friends and family that carried us through. (Since it was Communion weekend and I wasn't at church, people found out about our concerns.) I didn't trust going anywhere under the circumstances.

One night when I lay awake, it suddenly dawned on me, "I'm pregnant!" A happy feeling engulfed me despite our fears. I wanted to cling to this joyous sensation and not let it out of my grasp. For so long, we'd prayed for this and it had finally happened!

Monday morning dawned, at long last. Around 8:00 I began spotting, which came as no surprise. I'd been expecting it to happen at any minute. About an hour later, we left for the hospital and dropped off the boys at my parents, not knowing how long it would be till we'd see them again.

I was scheduled for a transvaginal ultrasound, which meant, thankfully, that I didn't need to endure a full bladder.

After another stressful wait at the hospital, it was finally our turn to be called. Our hearts sank when we saw who the technician was—the same grumpy guy who'd done the ultrasound in the spring. I felt like crying. Would we again be told to "not talk" when we so badly wanted to know?

Thankfully, this time he was much friendlier. (Was it because he was not working overtime this round?) Presently, he showed us a dark object (our baby!) in the uterus! Thank God! Our hearts overflowed with thanksgiving and relief. How good God was!

Our baby was indeed in the uterus, but there was a lot of extra blood. We knew our baby had no chance. The flickers of the tiny heartbeat showed on the screen, and oh, how we cherish that memory! It is the only memory of our dear baby.

We left the hospital and picked up our boys, happy that no surgery was needed. Several hours later, our precious baby left this earth, only four hours after we'd seen the heartbeat. The date was October 23, the very day our other baby would have been due. Instead of a precious baby to love and cherish, our second little one went to join the angels. It was a bittersweet day—a day of many emotions jumbled together.

Another special memory of this day was the one, lone, pure white (with a pink center) blossom on our Christmas cactus. It seemed Heaven-sent, like God was reminding us of His loving presence. The pure whiteness of the blossom depicted the innocent purity of our precious babies, safe in the arms of Jesus.

I think it is such a blessing that both times we were spared the anticipation of a baby, only to have our hopes dashed to pieces. I thank God for this wonderful blessing. Each time, by the time we discovered I was pregnant, we knew there was something wrong, and had no chance for getting our hopes high.

I have discovered the most difficult part of losing an unborn baby is the time when other women come to church with their babies who are the age ours would be. Oh, the longing to hold our precious baby! I hug my big two-year-old to myself and wish he weren't in such a big hurry to grow up.

I am so grateful for the gift of wonderful friends, who have worn the same difficult shoes, with whom we can share our fears, worries and hopes. In our church two more women had ectopics after mine (all three of ours happening in the space of nine months). We can truly feel for each other and it is encouraging to know we are not the only "oddballs."

A song that became one of my favorites is:

"When burdens come so hard to bear,
That no earthly friend can share,
Tears drive away the smiles and leave my heart in pain.
Then my Lord from Heaven above,
Speaks to me in tones of love;
Wipes the tears away and makes me smile again.

I need no mansion here below,
For Jesus said that I could go,
To a home beyond the clouds not made with hands.
Won't you come and go along?
We will sing the sweetest song
Ever played upon the harps in glory land."

We do not know what the future holds, but we know Who holds the future. We trust He will not give us more than He is willing to help us bear. We have been blessed with so much.

"Gathering flowers for the Master's bouquet,
Beautiful flowers that will never decay,
Gathered by angels and carried away,
Forever to bloom in the Master's bouquet."

Beloved, the next time you feel the heat of a fiery trial, thank God. It is proof of your preciousness to Him. You are His blood-bought child; you belong to Him; you may be sure that He cares for His own.

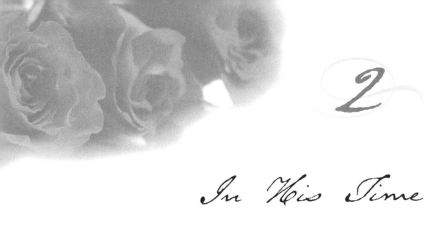

In His Time

—*Andrew & Shirley Martin, Alma, ON*

FRIDAY, SEPTEMBER 8, 2006, started out like many other days in our household. My husband, Andrew, went to work around 7:30 a.m. After two years of marriage, we were quite accustomed to this schedule. As usual, our one-year-old son, Jamie, was wide awake and ready to start his day too.

I was glad to get an early start on my day's work, as I wanted to can a batch of vegetable soup. I was busy preparing vegetables and meat for the jars of soup when, about mid-morning, I started feeling minor cramping, similar to menstrual cramps. I discovered that I was spotting a bit. I had some spotting the day before too, but now it was getting heavier. I knew it was too soon for me to be getting my period, so of course these signs raised a few questions in my mind. I decided I would call my doctor's office and see what I should do. I wasn't too keen on leaving my canning half done, but I decided that if I didn't call, I would have to wait until Monday. Not knowing what the weekend would bring, it seemed best to call the office. I talked with one of the nurses and explained my problem. When she heard that I had just recently stopped nursing Jamie, she said she thinks that my body is just getting back into its cycle after having nursed a baby. She told me not to worry.

I went back to my canning, relieved that I wouldn't have to

bother seeing the doctor, since I didn't feel I had time for that. In the back of my mind, though, I questioned the explanation I had been given. I had been having my period quite regularly for several months, and it seemed strange for my body to be acting like this. However, I didn't dwell on it, and went on with my day's work.

That afternoon, as I sat at the sewing machine, I started having more painful cramps. I soon felt too bad to be sewing at all, so I curled up on the couch with a book. Jamie played happily with his toys as I lay on the couch, trying to read and cope with the ever-worsening pain. It was like a giant hand squeezing my insides, and, in fact, reminded me very much of what it felt like to be in labor. After an hour of agonizing pain that was spreading from my lower right side to my back, I decided to call Andrew at work. It was 5:30, and I knew he'd be home in an hour, but at that point, an hour seemed like forever. I didn't know if I could manage that long.

I felt rather foolish calling Andrew and asking him to leave a half hour early, but I did. He sounded rather bewildered too, but after hearing my story, he promised, "I'll be home soon." Just having talked to him made me feel better, but the pain was still very intense. I wrapped an ice pack in a towel and pressed it against my back. It offered some relief. Again, I thought of when I had been in labor with Jamie and had done the same thing. "If I were pregnant, I'd think I *am* in labor," I thought wryly. But I knew that was not possible, as I'd just had my period one and a half weeks before.

Andrew came home shortly before 6:00. The pain had lessened slightly, and suddenly a trip to the emergency room didn't seem necessary. After all, the nurse had given me an explanation for my symptoms, and (I convinced myself) the pain wasn't that bad anymore. I certainly didn't want to look foolish, coming into the ER because of a few minor cramps! We debated about what we should do, and finally Andrew suggested that I take a hot bath, a cure for anything in his mind! I did so, while he got some supper for Jamie and himself. After my hot soak, I truly felt much better, but I still thought maybe I should get myself checked out. After discussing it with Andrew, we decided it was best to at least call the ER.

"Hello, Palmerston Hospital, Emergency Room." As I explained why I was calling, I felt a little foolish again, especially when I was told that the ER staff are not to give out medical advice over the phone. However, the receptionist listened to my story, and then she asked if the pain was bearable.

"Yes, I can handle it," I said stoically, thinking, *At least NOW I can! I almost couldn't a few hours ago!*

In that case, she told me, it would not be considered an emergency, but only something to be dealt with at the doctor's office during regular hours. "But," she cautioned, "if there is any possibility that you are pregnant, it would be an entirely different story."

> Those hard situations are put into your lives to change you. Stop praying for them to change, but pray that they may change you. —H. Markham

I quickly assured her that I was most definitely not pregnant, and after telling her I was pretty sure I could handle the pain, we hung up.

The rest of the evening was spent in a relaxing manner, and by bedtime, I could honestly feel no pain. I was so glad we hadn't gone to the ER; I would have felt so foolish! I crawled into bed, ready to forget the day's happenings, and naively believing all was well.

The next morning was Saturday. As soon as I awoke, I knew that all was *not* well. I had stomach pains again, though not nearly as bad as on Friday. The pain was a constant pressure in my abdomen. It was like a huge weight sitting in my stomach. When I leaned forward, it "rolled" forward, when I lay on my side, the pressure moved there. The pain was bearable most of the time, but as I slowly moved about my work, it would occasionally get very intense. I would quickly sit down, and in a few seconds, it would subside again, and I would keep going. I was growing more worried, too, and as my thoughts roamed, I had to tell myself over and over that God was still in control, and would provide strength for whatever we would face.

I ate only a few mouthfuls all day, and only because I forced myself to. I felt as if I had just eaten a big chicken dinner, but I knew it wasn't a full stomach that made me feel so bloated. I took frequent breaks from my work that day, and spent a lot of time on the couch, poring over our out-of-date medical books. I saw the list of symptoms for a tubal pregnancy several times, and I did have several of the symptons, but always I thought it to be impossible. Sometimes doubts nagged in the back of my mind, but I always dismissed them with the same reasoning; I couldn't possibly have conceived since my last period, so a tubal pregnancy wasn't possible either.

By Saturday evening, I was quite convinced that whatever was wrong with me was not just a minor thing. I counted the hours until Monday, when I could see my doctor, but even so, I didn't really believe that I would be sent home with a bottle of pills that would cure my problem. I just had a feeling it was more extensive than that, but only God knew what the next week would bring, and until then, we could only trust in Him.

On Sunday we had Communion services at church. I went,

still feeling full, bloated and miserable. I didn't get a lot out of the service, though, as my mind was occupied with coping with my pain. We spent the rest of the day at home, Andrew reading and me worrying. Again I studied our medical book and considered the possibilities. Ovarian cysts? Tubal pregnancy? Cancer? None of these prospects looked very bright. I wished I could be more like Andrew, who didn't bother worrying. His outlook was, "Whatever happens, happens." I, on the other hand, was too impatient to just wait it out; I wanted to try and figure out what was going on. But I kept reminding myself that I must leave things in God's hands.

Over the whole weekend, as I became more and more convinced of something seriously wrong, I spent much time playing with Jamie. He was 14 months old, and so very precious to us! Just recently I had started dreaming of how it would be to have another baby. I was eager to be pregnant again, but I also wanted to enjoy the son God had given to us. As I played with him, I wondered who would take care of Jamie if I had to spend time in a hospital. But I quickly turned off these thoughts, scolded myself for assuming the worst and focused on enjoying the present.

Monday morning finally came. I was still feeling bloated and cramped, and, since I'd barely had any solid food on Sunday, it was obvious that something was wrong. At 8:30 sharp, I was on the phone, calling the doctor's office. I desperately hoped to see my own family doctor, and what a relief—she was in that day! I had an appointment at 2:00, which couldn't come soon enough for me.

As the day progressed, the pain started to lessen somewhat. I was feeling better than I had at any time since Friday night, but after my miserable weekend, I knew I still wanted to see my doctor. My mom gladly agreed to baby-sit Jamie, so after taking him there, I headed for the doctor's office.

As I sat in the waiting room, I thought about the date: September 11. It sounded so ominous, being so securely linked to the terrorist attacks of 2001. I wondered if the date would hold new meaning for us too. I was prepared to receive bad news, or at least warnings of possible bad news, but again, I wanted to leave everything to God.

My name was finally called, and I went into the examining room with the nurse. She asked me different questions: the nature of the pain, when it started, when I had my last period, whether it was normal or not, when I quit nursing Jamie, etc. I answered them all as best as I could, and soon my doctor came in. She went over the same questions, and then asked me to lie on the examining table. As I lay down, she asked me, "Is there anything in particular that you have been worrying about recently? Any big stresses in your life right now?"

"Well, this," I said, half jokingly, pointing to my stomach.

"Is there anything you are particularly worried that it might be? I might be able to assure you about some things that it's not," she replied, genuinely concerned.

It crossed my mind to blurt out "tubal pregnancy," but I was still convinced I couldn't be pregnant, and I knew she knew I'd had my period only one and a half weeks ago, so I didn't say anything. As the doctor poked and prodded my stomach, I didn't flinch. It didn't really hurt much, but I thought to myself, *If you'd have done that on Saturday, I would have screamed!* But for some reason, my pain was just not as intense anymore. She asked if her prodding was giving me pain, and I answered, "A little, but not much." I definitely didn't want to make things sound worse than what they were.

After a short examination, my doctor gave me her opinion. She believed my bleeding was due to my period being regulated after weaning my baby. The pain was not related to that, but was due to ovulation, as it was almost two weeks since my last period. I took this all in without expressing what I was feeling in any way. As soon as I heard her diagnosis, I already doubted its accuracy, but I made no comment. She continued, "However, just to be safe, we'll have you book an ultrasound at the hospital, to make sure you don't have ovarian cysts or something similar. I'll get you the requisition, and you can call the hospital and book it when you get home. Or, if you like, you can wait until tomorrow. If you are feeling better, you don't have to get an ultrasound done at all." I nodded, trying to make it appear as if I believed what she said. But inside, my mind was whirling. I had been prepared to hear much, much worse news, and this seemed like such an oversimplified answer to my problem! I didn't argue of course; I just got my requisition papers and left. But when I came out of the office, I started listing all the reasons that made me think she was wrong.

The fact that my doctor didn't insist on an ultrasound told me that she didn't think my problem was very serious. I appreciated and respected her very much, but I just wasn't satisfied with this diagnosis. I couldn't convince myself that all my pain and bleeding weren't related at all, nor did I believe that ovulation could bring on such intense pain. Besides all that, my pride was a little injured too! I didn't want to look like someone who ran to the doctor for every little ache and pain, and that's exactly what my doctor made me feel like. But there wasn't much I could do at that point. I did book an ultrasound as soon as I got home. I decided that even if nothing showed up, at least I would have peace of mind. My ultrasound appointment wasn't until two days later, on Wednesday afternoon.

On Tuesday I was feeling even better than before, and as I energetically canned pizza sauce and ketchup, I was slowly starting to change my opinion about my doctor's diagnosis. She had predicted that both the pain and the bleeding would subside and disappear in the next few days, and it appeared she was right on both points. I began to feel ridiculous about my ultrasound appointment, too. Was I just desperate for attention, doing all this doctoring when there was nothing wrong with me?

Since my symptoms had pretty much disappeared, I didn't think much about my ultrasound appointment. Andrew fully believed what the doctor had told me, and by Tuesday evening I was pretty much convinced, too. I supposed that I would still get an ultrasound done, and probably in a few days I'd get a phone call from the doctor's office, saying all was well. After that, I thought, life would go on as before.

Wednesday, September 13, 2006, started very early for me. Around 3:00 a.m. Jamie woke up, as some of his teeth were bothering him. As soon as I awoke, I realized that the painful, bloated feeling was back, as intense as ever. I also noticed that I was bleeding again. (This had completely stopped sometime on Tuesday.) When I discovered that, I knew instantly that my doctor *was* wrong. The pain and bleeding *had* to be connected somehow, if they both started at the same time. As I paced the floor with Jamie in the wee hours, I thought with relief of my ultrasound appointment for the next day. I was ready to find out the cause of my ailments, once and for all.

Jamie didn't settle down again until 6:00, so Andrew and I got one more hour of sleep. Neither of us had slept much between 3:00 and 6:00, so we were not exactly well rested as we got up to start the day. Little did we know that we wouldn't see our bed again for 21 hours!

Wednesday morning passed uneventfully enough. I puttered around the house, not doing much, just waiting for the time to pass. I did not feel very well, and because of my bloated feeling I was back to a liquids-only diet. This turned out to be a blessing later in the day! At 12:30, I had to drink four cups of liquid in preparation for my ultrasound. I could hardly bear the thought of having so much in my stomach at one time, but I managed to drink it. Needless to say, though, I didn't eat any lunch!

At 1:30 I sat in the waiting room at the hospital, hoping that no one familiar would see me. They would, of course, think I was pregnant, but I *wasn't*! I was soon called into the ultrasound room. It seemed quite familiar, since I had several ultrasounds done during my first pregnancy, but this time was definitely different—something was *wrong* with me.

It was only a minute or two into the ultrasound when the radiologist asked me when my last period was. I told her it had been two weeks before, and she asked if there had been anything unusual about it. I said no, and then remembered one thing.

"Well, I did have a bad backache, kind of like I did when I was pregnant," I told her.

"Oh, really? At the beginning or at the end of your pregnancy?" She seemed very interested to know.

"The beginning," I answered, carefully watching her face for any hint of what she might be thinking.

"Hmm," was her only response. Then she asked, "And have you been using any sort of birth control?"

Instantly all the red flags were waving in my mind. *She wouldn't ask that unless there was some possibility of my being pregnant! And she was doing an ultrasound after all. What better way to tell if I was pregnant or not?*

"Does it look like I'm pregnant?" I responded, my voice much more calm than what I felt.

"Well, there's something funny going on here," was her reply. There was another brief pause, then she asked, "Do you know what a tubal pregnancy is?"

"Sort of," I answered. "But explain it to me anyway."

"I haven't found anything yet, so we won't go there," she replied, evading my request. After several more minutes of probing, she said, "We're going to have to do a pregnancy test. If it is positive, that will probably mean a tubal pregnancy, since there's nothing in your uterus. That is considered a medical emergency, which means it would have to be taken care of today, through surgery. And even if you aren't pregnant, we will need to do a more extensive ultrasound to find out what is causing your pain and bleeding."

I was in a sort of daze as I got up from the bed and followed her to the hospital lab. *This is impossible. I can't be pregnant,*" my mind insisted, but that voice was fading out as reality set in. *They wouldn't do a pregnancy test if it weren't a possibility,*" I argued. The blood test took only a few minutes, but the results would take half an hour or longer. I was sent back to the waiting room to do just that—wait.

The next 45 minutes were probably the longest of my life. I sat and flipped through magazines, studiously looking at each article, yet not comprehending a thing I read. The probability of a pregnancy was suddenly very real. I had spent the last five days telling myself it wasn't possible, so I was in a state of confusion and apprehension. Every few minutes I would look at the clock: 2:17....2:28....2:35.... The minutes crept by while I waited and prayed in the waiting room, wishing Andrew was there with me. Outwardly, I was as cool and calm as everyone else in the room, but that belied the turmoil inside me.

Finally, after a three-quarter hour wait, the radiologist called me into her room again. "The test was positive," she said kindly. "You are pregnant." Even though I had spent the last hour preparing myself for this possibility, the words came as a shock. I listened with only one ear as she explained the next procedure, an internal ultrasound. As I lay down again, I was thinking, *This isn't how it's supposed to feel when you find out you're pregnant. That should be a joyful time, not like this.* I wasn't even sure how I felt, just simply very empty and numb with shock. At any rate, I had no hopes of seeing this baby carried to full term. I was now quite certain that this must be a tubal pregnancy, and I started preparing myself for that verdict. The radiologist interrupted my thoughts. "How often have you been pregnant?" she asked.

"Once," I answered firmly.

She smiled. "You mean twice."

I smiled too. "Yeah, I guess I have to get used to this."

After a few more minutes of silence, she wondered, "So where is your husband?"

"He's at work," I replied, immediately sensing that she was trying to prepare me for bad news. "Should he be here?"

"Well, we won't worry yet. I haven't found anything." She continued moving her probe, and only a few more minutes had passed when she suddenly said, "Oh-oh, I think I found the problem." Turning the screen toward me, she pointed to a red ring on the screen. "This is what we look for in a tubal pregnancy," she explained. "It is very evident, so I think we can be assured that is the problem." She then pointed to a big black mass on the screen. "That's all fluid in your abdomen," she explained. "Are you in a lot of pain?" I honestly replied that, no, I wasn't. I definitely had a pressure in my stomach, but it wasn't very intense pain at all. She chuckled, "Well, you should be." Inwardly I thanked God that He had spared me from the intense pain I should have felt.

The radiologist then left the room to call my family doctor, and let her know what was happening, and I was left perched on the edge of the bed, lost in my thoughts. So that was it. I was pregnant, but they would take my baby away. I was in too much shock to feel any sadness right then. The knowledge that I was pregnant had hardly hit me yet, so knowing that I would be losing a baby was incomprehensible to me. I just felt very matter-of-fact about the whole issue.

The radiologist came back and explained that I would need to be transferred to Stratford Hospital, about an hour's drive away, for my surgery. She also said that my doctor wanted to talk to me on the phone. I was very relieved, as I had been feeling a little overwhelmed, and to have my own doctor talk to me made me feel less like just a statistic, and more like a person who was under her medical care.

"Hello, Shirley. How are you?" came my doctor's soft voice on the phone. I almost blurted out "fine" before I realized how silly that would sound, considering the circumstances, so I just said, "I'm okay." She proceeded to apologize for misdiagnosing me on Monday. A tubal pregnancy had come to her mind, but she thought it wasn't a possibility since I'd just had a period. I assured her that I had used exactly the same reasoning to rule out a tubal pregnancy. Then she told me what to expect when I got to Stratford. I assured her that Andrew would be able to take me there right away, and that we could make arrangements for Jamie to stay somewhere, possibly for a few days, while I was in the hospital.

After I was done talking with her, I called Andrew at work to tell him about the afternoon's events. He was quite unprepared for that, as he had also assumed I wouldn't get a report that day. He promised to leave work right away, pick up some clothes and personal belongings at home for me, then come to the hospital. Next I called my mom and told her what was going on. I knew that between his two sets of grandparents, Jamie would be very well cared for.

After all the arrangements were made, the radiologist took me over to the emergency room. It was only then that I noticed she was pregnant. Inwardly I thought, *That's not fair! Why can you have a healthy pregnancy and I can't?* But she had taken very good care of me in a trying time, and I knew it wasn't her fault that I had a tubal pregnancy. She left me in the care of the ER nurses, and went on her way.

I waited for Andrew for another hour, dazedly flipping through magazines, and comprehending absolutely nothing that I read. I felt surprisingly relaxed and patient, although I did watch the clock quite closely. I knew I would have surgery sometime that day, but I had been so unprepared for the news that it hadn't completely registered in my mind. When Andrew finally came, I felt like throwing myself in his arms, but instead we just smiled and greeted each other with our customary dry, "Hi." The ER nurses gave us a hand-drawn map to show us where we were going, and sent us on our way.

The drive to Stratford was filled with lighthearted chatter between Andrew and me. I filled him in on the details of the afternoon's events, and he told me about his abrupt exit from work. I was thinking of the upcoming surgery, and it was not an appealing thought. I confided my dread to Andrew, and he sympathized, saying that he didn't blame me for not looking forward to it. It was probably best, though, that I hadn't had more time to worry about it.

We finally arrived at the emergency entrance to Stratford

Hospital. We soon realized that this was no light-flashing, sirens-blaring emergency like I had imagined. After we had done some paperwork to admit me to the hospital, we sat in the waiting room for half an hour. Then I was taken to a private room, where I put on a hospital gown and climbed into bed. I was starting to feel like a sick person, but just because I was in bed, not because I was ill! Physically, I was feeling very close to normal again, so it was kind of hard to believe that my condition was considered a medical emergency.

It was around 5:30 when we arrived at the hospital, and in total, we spent four and a half hours just waiting until there was finally an opening for me in the operating room. Andrew and I sat and visited lightheartedly, too much in shock and too tired to have any deep philosophical conversations. Occasionally, though, I would wistfully say, "I'm pregnant! Oh, I wish we could keep this baby!" But we both knew that was impossible. The hours slowly crept by. Every time a nurse or doctor came in, we hoped they would take me to surgery. But they would only check up on me, start an IV, bring some more forms to fill out, ask more questions, etc. One nurse informed us that since there were no empty rooms in the hospital, I would need to go home that night, after my surgery. As more time passed, we realized that this was going to be a long, long day.

Around 8:00 the surgeon came in to meet us, and to explain the procedure he would use. He would perform a laparoscopy, which involved inserting a scope just below my navel. This allowed him to see what was going on. He said he would try to salvage my tube, but if it was too badly damaged, he would remove it, rather than having another tubal pregnancy later because of a defective tube. I was still confused about why I had a period just two weeks before, so I asked him if there's any possible way to tell when I had conceived. He said it had to be the cycle before my last period, which would have put my pregnancy about six weeks along. He said it was common for tubal pregnancies to act up around that mark, so it was a reasonable estimate.

We waited for another two hours, until finally, at 10:00, I was taken to the operating room. I was so tired and cold, and I was not impressed when my wheelchair was simply parked in the hallway for another half hour. As I watched the nurses bustling in and out of the rooms, I thought back over the last eight hours, and I could hardly fathom what had all happened. My 2:00 ultrasound appointment in Palmerston Hospital seemed like days ago!

At last they wheeled me into the operating room. I had been asked many times that day if I had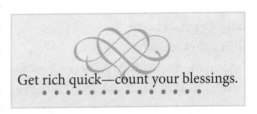

Get rich quick—count your blessings.

anything to eat, and fortunately for me, I'd only had liquids. That was a good way to go into surgery! The one nurse explained that they would inject a gas into my abdomen to make everything more accessible. "But," he warned, "it can make you very, very nauseated. We'll give you medication for that, but," he shook his head, "it's really nasty stuff." I had been hoping my surgery wouldn't be as bad as I had imagined, but at that point I simply resigned myself to being sick afterward.

Soon my chest was plastered with monitors and wires. Then I was warned that the anesthesia was being administered, and a few seconds later, my eyes grew heavy, and blackness engulfed me.

My surgery lasted one hour. When my surgeon opened me up, he had pretty high hopes of salvaging my tube. It had not actually ruptured, but there was a lot of bleeding already, and he soon gave up on the idea of saving it. All that blood and other fluid in my abdomen explained the "full" feeling I had been having. He removed the tube, and sewed me up again.

Around midnight I woke up fully, and soon a nurse was by my side. I remembered exactly what was happening, and why I had surgery. I asked her if my tube had been removed. She said it had, and that was all I needed to know just then. I didn't feel any strong emotions on hearing that; I had just been curious. Andrew came into the room then, and I was very glad to see him. Thankfully, he had been able to sleep some in the waiting room. I knew he was tired after having so little sleep the night before, and now he had to drive for an hour to get us home.

At 2:00 a.m., after two hours of "recovery," the nurse kindly helped me get ready to go home. I sat up, waiting for waves of nausea to wash over me, but they never came. Miraculously, I was completely spared from any nausea! I took a painkiller, and the nurse bandaged my three small incisions, each only about one-half inch long. After I was dressed, the nurse wheeled me down the hall, and Andrew carried my bag. All the things I had brought with me in preparation for several days at the hospital weren't needed after all, but I didn't mind. Physically, I felt very well, and was eager to get home to my own bed, even at this hour.

It was 2:45 a.m. when we left the parking lot. As we drove out of the city. I asked Andrew, "Do you think we have a baby in Heaven now?" He said he didn't know, but we found it comforting to believe that way. We arrived home at 3:45 a.m. and crashed into our own bed. It was probably the longest, most emotionally exhausting day of our short married life!

I had many questions to ask the surgeon and my family

doctor. Neither of them could give a satisfactory explanation about why I had a period even when I was pregnant. But in doing some research on my own, I learned that one in four women continue to menstruate during a tubal pregnancy. I also sometimes wonder why my pain was so intense one day, and gone the next, and exactly what was going on when I had an hour or two of very severe pain on the first day. However, we have left it all in God's hands, and are just thankful that my condition wasn't worse by the time it was diagnosed.

Physically, I recovered very well from my surgery. My teenage sister-in-law helped us out for one week afterward, and from then on I easily managed the housework. I didn't feel that I suffered at all from loss of blood, and my three tiny incisions healed up very nicely.

Emotionally, however, it took more time to heal. The first morning after my surgery, reality had not set in yet. I opened my Bible to read, and David's Psalms of praise were the first that jumped out at me. I had so much to be thankful for: good health care, kind nurses, no nausea, a supportive husband, and a dear, sweet son to come home to. But by the end of that day, stark reality hit me, and I shed tears for the tiny life that was lost.

Throughout the next several weeks, I struggled with knowing whether my grief was "valid." Before this happened, I wouldn't have believed that you would need to grieve for a baby which was taken from you, when you had learned a mere eight hours previous that it even existed. But that is how our experience was, and we did grieve. Many people inquired about how I was feeling physically, and I always answered positively, as I had very little to recover from. But I was extremely grateful for anyone who also mentioned the loss of our baby, not just my surgery. Even though we hadn't known about the pregnancy yet, it was still a loss, and when people acknowledged this, I was thankful that they realized that I had not just had a body part removed, but a tiny life.

In the following weeks, I also battled with the knowledge that I had been pregnant for several weeks, but had never had the privilege of enjoying that secret with my husband. I knew I had been spared from having my dreams shattered, but I also felt as if I had been deprived of the joys of pregnancy, even of having dreams for our baby.

Family and friends reached out to us in many different ways, all of which were appreciated, and helped us cope. I also found it was important to keep busy. Sewing projects that I had only thought about became reality as I struggled through my grief. I threw myself into my housework, and perhaps most of all, into being a mom to dear little Jamie. His presence was very healing, as he was an ever-present reminder of God's goodness. We learned to be much more grateful for the gift of a healthy son, and we enjoyed him in a new and precious way.

There were some nights that I couldn't sleep, and so I would get up and write in my journal. I also wrote a detailed account of our experience. Both of these things were very therapeutic for me. I felt that we didn't have anything tangible to remember our baby by, so the next week, I cut a rosebud and dried it, in memory of this tiny life. I also decorated a box to put all our cards, letters and other mementos in, for a remembrance.

A passage of Scripture that became precious to me was Ecclesiastes 3:11.

"He hath made every thing beautiful in his time."

I also found comfort in Psalm 139:15 and 16.

"My substance was not hid from thee, when I was made in secret, and curiously wrought in the lowest parts of the earth. Thine eyes did see my substance, yet being imperfect; and in thy book all my members were written, which in continuance were fashioned, when as yet there was none of them."

This passage gave me assurance that God had been in control of this tiny life, and what had happened to it was all part of His plan. In the next weeks and months, as I saw others enjoying new babies, or hearing of others who were expecting babies, I also found the song "Thy Will Be Done" (#390, *Christian Hymnal*) to be very precious to me, especially the fourth verse:

"Renew my will from day to day,
Blend it with Thine, and take away,
All now that makes it hard to say,
Thy will be done."

Having a tubal pregnancy was a traumatic experience, but we thank God for bringing us through with a minimum of physical difficulties, and also for His comfort and healing as we grieved afterward. May He be the same Source of comfort for others who go through the same type of trial.

Stay firm; God has not failed thee
In all thy past,
And will He go and leave thee
To sink at last?
Nay, He said He will hide thee
Beneath His wing;
And sweetly there in safety
Thou mayest sing.

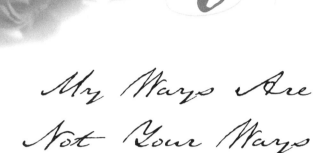

My Ways Are Not Your Ways

—*Brad & Gail Carter, Dalton, OH*

SEPTEMBER 9, 2004, started out like any other day. Little did we know what God had in store for us. My husband Brad left in the morning to teach school. I was planning to meet him around 2:00 that afternoon so we could leave for a doctor's appointment. I had been bleeding for several days, and I knew it couldn't be my period because I'd just had that a couple weeks before. But this bleeding acted like a period, too. At the time we were doctoring for infertility, so of course they wanted to check this bleeding out.

Around 1:00 that afternoon I was getting ready to go to the doctor, when all at once I had terrible pressure in my stomach. I became light-headed, so I lay on the couch. I soon thought I was okay, so I got up and took a bath. I felt awful pressure when I was in the tub. I then lay on the bed. Once I had gotten dressed I took a few things out to the car.

All at once I realized I was about to pass out... Quickly I got to the house, grabbed the phone and lay on the couch. I quickly called Brad and told him to come right away, as something is wrong, but I don't know what. He soon arrived—what a relief!

We tried to decide if we should just go to the closest hospital, or drive the 1 1/4 hours to Luther Hospital where we had been doctoring for infertility. We called down to Luther, and they wondered if we could come, since they had all my records.

I had to wonder how I'd make the trip with such extreme pain. We got into the car and started off, only to run into some road construction. Between that and stopping a couple of times to use the restroom, we kept pressing on. The pain had let up, but now I was terribly tired. I knew I had to stay awake, though.

Finally, two hours later we arrived at Luther Hospital. We got into the clinic and took the elevator up to the second floor. The doctor took us in right away, and started checking me by touching my stomach and checking my ovaries. It was *terribly* painful—words can't even describe it.

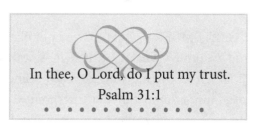

In thee, O Lord, do I put my trust.
Psalm 31:1

Nurses were soon drawing blood to take a pregnancy test. One test took only half an hour to get results. The other one, a more detailed one, would take two hours. In the meantime they kept checking me. Another thing they did was an ultrasound. It puzzled them because there seemed to be a big mass of something.

They quickly called for Dr. Burgess to come. By this time the room was getting rather full with nurses and doctors. Suddenly fear struck—whatever was wrong with me? I tried to relax and lean on the Lord. Soon the results from the quick pregnancy test came back, saying I was pregnant. I could hardly believe it; I had no idea I was pregnant.

Dr. Burgess was soon saying, "I'm taking you to surgery!"

She thought it might be a tubal, but wasn't 100% sure, since the blood work wasn't back yet. We went back to my original room where Dr. Burgess met with us and quickly went over the details of the surgery. Then we signed the papers for the go-ahead. It was an awful blow when she looked at me and said, "This is a life-threatening surgery." I can't explain the feeling that went through me.

The lab lady soon came in to draw more blood, then I changed into a gown for surgery.

Brad and I spent a minute together before I went for surgery. I kept wondering, "Will I make it through?" Brad tried to reassure me. We cried and prayed together. Soon they were at the door, wanting to take me over to the hospital. I got into the wheelchair and they pushed me over. By then the pain was up in my chest. It felt like someone was stabbing me with a butcher knife.

They got me ready for surgery. Brad called home to his folks and told them what was going on. We had left in such a hurry that no one knew what had happened. Then he got hold of my parents in Ohio, some seven hundred miles away.

Soon they were ready to take me into the operating room. Brad could only follow till the big doors came into view. Then we said, "Good-bye." It was an awfully hard parting, the uncertainty of not knowing if I'd ever see my wonderful husband again. Tears brimmed my eyes. I started to cry, but pain shot into my chest.

They pushed the bed into the surgery room, then took both ends of the sheet and lifted me up on the operating table. I couldn't move without the killing pain hitting me. They soon finished hooking me up to more IVs. Soon the anesthesia started working. I remember looking at the clock and it was 7:00. So much had happened in two and a half hours since we had arrived at the hospital. They told me that the two-hour blood test had come back, saying it was a ruptured tubal pregnancy, but I don't remember anyone telling me this. I must have been just going to sleep.

Next thing I knew a nurse was at my side, wondering how I felt. I tried to see her, but my eyes just would not focus. I told her that I still have bad pain. She assured me that they were going to hook me up to morphine. I awoke again to find Brad by my side. This time my vision was clear. I noticed it was after 9:00. I had been in surgery for two hours. It had been a major surgery! I had a five-inch incision, where they had opened me up and stitched the right tube back together.

My sharp pain had come from bleeding internally and by that time I was filled up to my ribs with blood. They told me there were huge clots. They pulled the clots out and rinsed me out a couple times, by putting water in and tipping me back and forth to get all the stuff washed out. I had lost lots of blood and was right at the point of needing blood. But they felt I was young enough that I'd work back my blood, so they didn't give me any.

They pushed my bed out of the recovery room and put it on the elevator to take me to the second floor, where I had my own private room. Once I got off the elevator, I spied some of Brad's family. The nurses put me into my bed and got me situated. I felt so weak and tired. I was on the same floor as moms with babies. I remember thinking I'm so glad I don't have to take care of a baby yet. I didn't think I'd have the strength to do it. Deep down I knew I wanted a baby sometime—just not right then!

My mom flew up from Ohio on Saturday and helped me for several days. I was ordered to do almost nothing for six weeks. I was so tired and weak that for the first few weeks it wasn't even a temptation to get up and do hard work. The family, church people and friends helped me out after Mom left for home. We appreciated everyone's help.

I came home on Saturday. The following Tuesday we went back to get the nine staples taken out. I then asked Dr. Burgess some things I was wondering about and she explained everything. One thing I thought was interesting—on the way to the hospital I got so tired. She told me that it's awfully good that I didn't fall asleep, because with a ruptured tubal pregnancy, if you do fall asleep you probably wouldn't wake up again!

She also said once a tube has ruptured, the pain lets up for a little while, so sometimes people think it's not too serious, because the pain left. When in reality you are in a very serious condition. I asked her how far along in the pregnancy I was. She guessed about eight weeks. They told me if I ever get pregnant again, I have a 20% chance of having another tubal. They also informed me that a ruptured tubal pregnancy is the most painful thing to go through.

The days following were some very dark and dreary days. The reality of it all hit me while I was recuperating. The thought came to me that we had actually lost a baby. I often wondered, *Why did God spare my life?* I knew it wouldn't have been long before I would have been gone. God must still have a purpose for me in this life, and I want to be faithful to Him and fulfill that purpose.

I had a round of depression, which doctors told me is very common for people who have gone through serious surgeries. The Lord helped us through. I know the prayers of family and friends helped me through the dark valley. Psalm 139 became very dear to me. It was such a comfort to read that chapter and know that God is with us no matter where we are or what we are going through. Also, in the book of Job a verse says, "When He has tried me I shall come forth as gold." A song that often comes to mind is...

"Oft the way to the goal seems so weary and long,
Trials almost take away our song.
Then we sigh and we cry and we ask, Father, why
Does this life my wishes all deny?

Chorus:
My ways, my child, are not your ways,
My thoughts are higher than thine.
Let me lead you each step of this long, weary day,
Let me clasp thy trembling hand in mine."

In June of 2006, God blessed us with our first child—a little girl, whom we love and cherish very much. We did not know if we'd be able to have children or not. God answered our prayers. He has kept us thus far and we trust Him for the future.

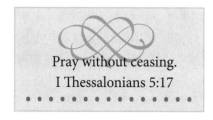

Pray without ceasing.
I Thessalonians 5:17

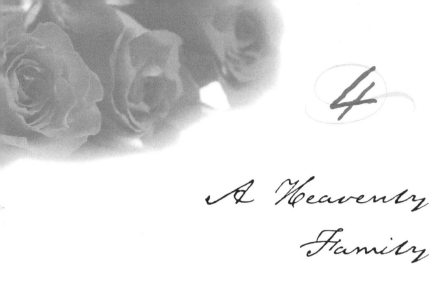

4

A Heavenly Family

—*Lowell & JoAnn Brenneman, Falkville, AL*

IN MAY OF 1991 a son arrived in our home to begin our family. Little did we realize what the next three and one half years held for us.

I started bleeding on December 20, 1991, and something about how I was feeling just didn't seem right. But I didn't know what was going on. I don't believe I even realized I was pregnant, but a test was taken, with a positive result. This was on a Friday.

Saturday afternoon a good friend of mine from Pennsylvania arrived. Soon after her arrival something was said that brought on laughter, which hurt my side so bad I covered my face with a pillow to hide my discomfort. (My pain during the day was off and on and quite severe.) After this experience I let Lowell, my husband, know that I was ready to see a doctor.

Dr. Inhulsen was willing to meet us at the office that Saturday afternoon. It took two people to help me to the car, but after arriving at the office I was able to walk unattended. One of the things he did was to push gently on my abdomen and then give a quick release. My reaction gave a good indication of internal bleeding. He sent us on to the hospital. Prior to being taken to the operating room I passed out for a short time.

The operation revealed a ruptured ectopic pregnancy in the left tube and a loss of one liter of blood. The tube had ruptured transversely. The area was cleaned up and felt to be useless as it was, so the doctor left it there.

The ride to the hospital was different in that I didn't know if the Lord would be calling me Home to Him. God has been good. The journey has not always been easy, but God has been faithful.

After the tubal, I experienced some miscarriages as well as a molar pregnancy in 1993. We did not know if the Lord would bless us with more children. With each episode it would just be that much longer before we'd have more children. We probably missed out on some blessings, and now I realize it is best to make the most of whatever God gives, whether it means being childless, or having any number of children. God has something for us all.

Following a normal pregnancy, a tubal pregnancy, several miscarriages and a molar pregnancy (after which they didn't want me pregnant for a year), I conceived again and gave birth to our second son. This was nearly four years after our firstborn.

In 1999 I experienced another tubal pregnancy in the partial left tube. I was quick to identify the pain. This time it was on a Sunday morning. We had moved from Georgia to Alabama since the time of the first tubal, but fortunately the midwife we had been working with on previous pregnancies knew a doctor that was willing to see us in his office that morning. We were transferred to the hospital and this time the tube was removed.

God has blessed us with a Heavenly family as well as an

earthly family. We are now looking forward to the arrival of our eighth child.

The miscarriages I've experienced are around 7 1/2 weeks, so about the time I start feeling sick from a pregnancy, it either terminates or else I experience morning sickness for a few months.

A summary of our history:

May 14, 1991—Floyd
Dec. 1991—tubal
several miscarriages
1993—molar pregnancy
April 24, 1995—Joel
miscarriage
Dec. 26, 1996—Lavern
miscarriage
Nov. 26, 1998—Marcus
1999—tubal
Sept. 13, 2000—Ruth
May 4, 2002—Rosemary
miscarriage
Jan. 8, 2005—Charity
miscarriage
Feb. 2007—?

Giving birth is a miracle from the Lord, and I believe He can open or close the womb as He wills. He knows best. For us He's given us a family; for others He may have something else special for them. May we be faithful to the calling He has for us. God is good!

In Time of Disappointment

As you face your recent disappointment
You may wonder why it happened so—
Why the thing you waited, longed and prayed for,
Now before your eager grasp must go.

Why your worthy dream must now be shattered
And your life be robbed of quiet peace.
Do not murmur; all things have a reason.
Trust in God, and you will find release.

Though just now God's purpose may be hidden,
His direction hard to understand,
He is yearning that you yield completely,
Lest you thwart the work that He has planned.

For all stubbornness, or grief protracted,
Any clinging to the hope now lost,
Is a hindrance to God's perfect pattern;
You will have to face sometime the cost.

But God's leading is hard to follow;
He will help you bear the heavy cross,
For He does not ask His child to suffer
Too much disappointment, pain or loss.

Well He knows the weight of every trouble;
He has shaped this burden just for you.
Walk in close communion with your Father,
And His grace will help you through.

—*Mrs. Silas Bowman*

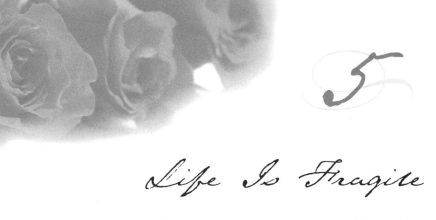

5

Life Is Fragile

—Harry & Barbara Bontrager, Haven, KS

LYING HELPLESSLY ON the stretcher inside the ambulance, I wondered what my family at home was doing. They didn't even know where I was. As far as they knew, I was in town to do some shopping, yet here I was, speeding toward the hospital, not knowing what lay ahead.

On that spring day, April 9, 2002, my family consisted of Harry, my husband of 14 years, and our four children: Jason (12), Carrie (10), James (5) and Austin (2). (Our third child, Deborah, had died at eight months old of severe heart defects seven years earlier.) Harry was 40 and I was 36. We lived on his home place, a dairy farm in the Amish community near Yoder, Kansas, next door to his widowed mother and two sisters, Mary and Anna.

As I had changed out of my chore clothes on Monday morning two weeks before, my stomach was hurting, so I lay down instead of eating breakfast. As I lay there, it seemed my pain was lower than my stomach, and soon I had such excruciating pain that I couldn't lie down or lean back, and could barely walk. I could not breathe deeply and had to sit with my head leaning forward or I had even worse pain shooting up my shoulders. I would cry out in pain if I tried to lean back.

Harry's sister, Anna, helped me finish dinner for his brother and nephew, who were there to help with the construction of our new free-stall barn. I was in distressing pain the rest of the day, and was so worn out from the pain and from having to stay in an upright position that I finally placed a chair in front of my recliner and rested my head on the chair back. That was how I spent the night. Harry slept on the couch, because he didn't know what was going on.

We had talked of going to the doctor that day, but I didn't know how I would do

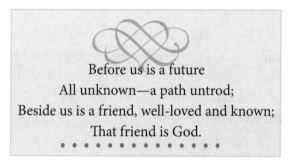

Before us is a future
All unknown—a path untrod;
Beside us is a friend, well-loved and known;
That friend is God.

it, since I could hardly move. I looked up everything from appendicitis to gallstones, but nothing matched my symptoms; I wasn't feverish or vomiting. I even looked up ectopic pregnancy, but felt certain that wasn't even a possibility, since I'd had a regular period just a little over two weeks earlier.

Toward morning I had a little relief and was able to lie back in the recliner. On Tuesday I still had much pain if I moved, but if I held perfectly still it wasn't too bad. So I thought I was getting better. That night I went upstairs to bed and was able to lie down, but it still hurt. When Harry came up, I told him I wish we would have gone to the doctor after all, just so we'd know what was going on.

So on Wednesday I got an appointment and went to town to see our family doctor. I was some better, but still moved slowly. The ride seemed rough, and my lower abdomen was very painful when pressed. I had noticed on Monday that my abdomen seemed so big. I told the doctor about all my symptoms, and he decided I had colitis, an inflammation of the colon, probably caused by a virus, and it should get better over the next few days. I told him about the pain in my shoulders, and he said because my colon was inflamed, it was pressing up against the diaphragm and caused referred pain in the shoulders. He wondered if I could be pregnant, but I told him I wasn't.

So home I went, happy that I was going to live after all. Each day I felt a little better, although I was still very weak, which I attributed to the pain and not eating for so long.

I read everything I could to learn more about colitis, and slowly started eating again, things like rice and vegetable gruel or bananas, hoping not to irritate this colon of mine. I also took food enzymes, in hopes I wouldn't have to live with such terrible gas pains again.

I thought I was getting along, until Friday morning at 2:00 a.m., when the pain started again. I moved down to my head-forward position on the recliner again, and had an exact replay of Monday. I was often in tears. It seems dumb now that we didn't go to the hospital then, but I thought I had this colitis and all the doctor had told me to do was take Pepto-Bismol, so I thought I'd have to live with it.

On Saturday morning we asked my sister-in-law to run to the herb shop in town to pick up aloe vera juice, "Intestinal Soothe and Build" capsules and magnesium (for the cramping), which was what they recommended for colitis when Harry called them. So I started swallowing that every few hours. By evening I did feel a little better. I spent the night on the recliner again and was still very weak on Sunday, but I felt delivered from the worst pain.

I moved slowly the next two days, but got around. We were supposed to have church services at our place in seven weeks, so I had that on my mind. On Wednesday morning I was still weak, but decided to wash and rinse the living room ceiling with the wall mop. I felt quite spent by the time I was finished. The next morning I did the dining room ceiling and thought I was stronger. Harry thought I should do just one ceiling a day, but I went ahead and did the small kitchen ceiling too, so I would be done. Then I did our porch ceiling yet, so I could forget about it, too.

By this time I was helping with the milking again in the evenings. On Friday I did our laundry, and thought it was hurting more. I always had such a heavy, uncomfortable feeling in my lower abdomen, and hurrying was out of the question. (When I'd had a second "attack," I did think to measure around my stomach, and a few days later, when I was "better," it was over two inches smaller.)

On Sunday, almost two weeks after my first pain, we were at our Communion services all day. I didn't really feel worse; I guess I was just kind of used to the constant discomfort and thought I have to live with this "colitis". At noon, I was not hungry at all, but did eat a half piece of bread.

On Tuesday afternoon, Allen Schrock took me to town to do some necessary shopping. Before I left, Anna came over to our house and asked if I'm going to see the doctor. I wondered what good that would do. Later she said I'd moved so slowly and looked so pale. Just that morning I had thought perhaps a chiropractor could help me, but I didn't make an appointment. Harry offered to make one for me, but I thought it would just take up more time. So off I went to town.

At my first stop, the discount store, I walked around with my cart, and all I could think about was how much I was hurting. I finally got some things and checked out. My next stop was at our county extension office, where I wanted to pick up a paper. I walked in very slowly. I sank onto a chair to wait while the lady went downstairs to fetch my paper on starting spring grass. I asked for their phone directory and copied my chiropractor's phone number. I went to the restroom and wondered what I shoud do. I didn't know if I should go home or what. I was in such pain, but was by myself, not knowing what to do.

I gave up my planned stops except for the grocery store. When I got there, I called the chiropractor's office for an appointment yet that afternoon. This was at 3:00 p.m. My regular doctor was full, but they said his partner could see me at 3:50. I went inside and got a big cart full of groceries. I got them out to the van and dragged myself back up into the front seat again. I still had books to drop off at the library, so we swung by the book drop box in the parking lot. I could hardly handle my big box full of books, but got it done and pulled myself back into the van.

As we headed for the chiropractor's office, I wondered what would happen if we'd just go to the medical center where my family doctor was located and tell them I have to see a doctor. But I didn't know if they'd want me dropping in unannounced. *What if there's nothing wrong with me??* So we drove right past the center and didn't stop.

I slowly, slowly walked in for my appointment, signed in and sat down to wait. After calling me back to the treatment room, the lady dutifully asked how I was doing. Then I fell apart and started crying and told her it hurts so bad and I don't even know if I should be there. Of course, she wasn't prepared for such a response, poor thing. I guess I wasn't either.

So she arranged for me to talk first with my regular chiropractor, saying he could see me in a little bit. She moved me into another room to wait, and shut the door. She stuck her head in a few times and I asked for a drink once. I was feeling worse and worse. I took off my apron and put it into my purse, because it was so painful under the belt. Then I took off my jacket. I felt clammy and cold and hot. I wondered if the doctor would never come. Finally, finally, after ten to fifteen minutes, the door opened and he came in. He asked me what's going on, and I wanted to tell him about colitis, but I couldn't seem to get it out.

The next thing I knew, I had a wet washcloth on my forehead, my feet were propped up, and he was telling me I had just passed out on him. (Later I found out I was out for five to ten minutes.) I managed to ask him if he could do anything for colitis.

He said, "Yes, but I think you need to see a doctor."

I wondered

Under his wings you will find refuge, and his faithfuless is a shield. Psalm 91:4

what I would do there, but halfheartedly agreed to go. He helped me to the door, and I walked slowly to the van and pulled myself in. I told Allen that he has to take me to the Medical Center and that I'd passed out in there. I could barely sit on the seat because every bump was excruciating. When we got there, I climbed the stairs by myself. Allen had offered to see about getting me a wheelchair, but I knew he couldn't manage it alone.

I walked in and told the receptionist that I have to see a doctor and that I had passed out. She disappeared and I sat down. Very soon the nurse came and took me to an exam room. She wanted to know what was going on, but before I told her much I gave her the telephone number of David and Annette, Harry's brother and wife, who lived down the road from us. She wanted me to get up on the exam table, but I took one look at it and knew I'd fall off that thing if I could even get on it.

I was starting to feel clammy again. She wanted me to put on a gown, but there was just no way I could, because of the pain. So I just sat on a chair. She took my temperature, but I had no fever.

She went to the door of my room, and I heard the doctor talking. She told him, "I can't leave her."

He said, "You can't leave her??" She repeated it again, so he came in and stood there and looked at me. "You mean you drop in here off the sidewalk, looking like this?!" I guess he wondered why I hadn't called before coming. I told him I had gotten worse while shopping.

They laid me on the exam table and he pressed around my abdomen a little bit. Almost at once he gravely told me, "You have to go to the hospital emergency room. There's something seriously wrong." I informed him that I'm in town alone. "You mean you drove by yourself in this shape?!" he exclaimed.

"Well, no," I said, "someone brought me in." I told them my driver is in the waiting room, but he said he doesn't want to send me that way. I didn't realize what the doctor knew: I had gone into shock and was bleeding internally.

He called 911, and it seemed like it was a few minutes later that I opened my eyes to see EMS-shirted guys putting an oxygen mask over my nose. I had my eyes closed most of the time and hardly knew what was going on. Then four of them picked me up and transferred me to the ambulance stretcher (OUCH), and rolled me out the door. They loaded me up, turned on the siren and headed for the hospital on the other side of town.

I was just barely "with it," but I remember thinking how absurd this was—here I'd gone shopping, now I'm in an ambulance, racing across town, and nobody knows I'm here. (They had told Allen to take my things home.) I had managed to ask if they'd call Harry, and I thought they said yes, but I knew he wasn't at home that afternoon and wondered how they'd find him. It was 5:00 p.m.

I felt very much alone, but could feel that God was with me through it all.

When I'd hear them discussing me, I kept hearing "suspect ectopic pregnancy." I kept thinking that can't be right.

After the initial rush at the emergency room, I was lying there alone, looking out at the team center, when the main P.A. who had examined me said to one of the others, "She is pregnant." I couldn't believe what I heard. The next time he came in I asked if he was talking about me and he said, "Yes." I asked how he knew, and he said they'd done a blood test at the doctor's office and the result was positive.

Now I didn't know what would happen. I had hoped and hoped that I wasn't pregnant so that whatever was wrong with me wouldn't endanger that, but now I knew it wasn't so.

Next they told me they're going to put in a catheter and take me for a sonogram. I wondered why I needed a catheter for that, since usually they want your bladder full. Well, they clamped it shut so it would get full, and later, in the ultrasound room, they even filled it up that way, by squeezing fluid in reverse through the tube.

It was just the technician and me for the next forty-five minutes or so. She didn't tell me what she sees and I didn't ask. I was just trying to endure the pain and hang on until Harry got there to hold my hand. They didn't want to give me any painkillers until they had a diagnosis.

I finally prayed that she wouldn't miss something like my appendix or gallbladder. At one point she asked me if I still have my gallbladder and when I had last eaten, so I thought, *Oh, it must be that.*

After they took me back to my ER spot at 7:15, the doctor came in and said the sonogram shows my abdomen is full of fluid, and most likely it is blood from a ruptured tubal pregnancy. They had called my OB doctor, and she soon arrived and explained everything to me. She said there was no sign of a pregnancy within the uterus, but that doesn't say there is none, and she would be very careful of that if she operates.

She said we could wait until morning and see what happens, but she wasn't comfortable with that and I wasn't either. She was really hesitant about doing anything without Harry there. Soon after that, Harry called and talked with her, so we decided to go ahead with surgery if they got ready before he could get there. This was certainly not the way I wanted it, but it seemed best under the circumstances. The OR staff said they could be ready in 20 minutes, so I was afraid I wouldn't get to see him. They took me in at 8:15, and he arrived 25 minutes later.

They used a laparoscope first, but soon had to go to a longer incision. She removed one tube and ovary; the ovary was also damaged. She said it was almost unrecognizable. The doctor said I had two liters of blood in there, and she had used liters and liters of water to flush it out.

One section of my colon was inflamed and matted against this ruptured mess, so she put in some kind of mat there to prevent scarring and adhesions. She told me later that she thinks perhaps this colon section had sometimes pressed against the bleeding and slowed it down enough that I would seem to get "better" between attacks of pain. She gave me one unit of blood to replace part of the large loss.

I woke up in the recovery room around 10:30. I heard Harry and sensed the black shape of his coat beside me. What a relief to have him there and holding my hand! One of the first things I asked him was, "What about having church in May?" I guess those female compulsions are hard to quench!

I came home three days later, and slowly recovered and regained my strength. Five weeks afterward, my incision became infected and I had to take a round of antibiotics.

We had a lot of "what-if?"s and "if only"s and "why?"s.

"If only" I had gone to the doctor on the first day I had the severe pain, maybe he wouldn't have let me off so easily. I have read that ectopic pregnancies are often misdiagnosed on the first visit. He was correct about the pressure on the diaphragm causing referred pain in the shoulders, but wrong about the cause, since it was blood instead of an inflamed colon.

"What if" I had passed out somewhere else in town and nobody would have known who I was??

"Why" did I have a regular period if I was pregnant? I had some spotting four or five days after my first attack, but since I hadn't missed a period, I didn't know what it meant. By not counting my last period, we estimated that I was probably at six weeks when my tube ruptured, according to the first signs.

When I think of everything I did, washing ceilings, milking, planting garden things, while bleeding internally, it makes me shudder. My doctor said I must have a very high pain tolerance to have made it so long. I don't know about that, but I thought all along that I was dealing with colitis.

Before she released me, my doctor warned me that if I ever become pregnant again it is imperative that I have a sonogram done as soon as I know, to rule out the possibility of another ectopic pregnancy. Having already had one will raise the risk of having another.

She told me that a woman's fertility with only one ovary is basically the same as with two. I don't know if others have found it so or not. I did not have any of the usual risk factors, such as endometriosis, pelvic inflammatory disease or cigarette smoking.

We were blessed with a baby girl thirteen months later, Katrina Joy. When Katrina was a little over three years old, we had another daughter born to us, Susanna Grace. Both pregnancies were normal. With both of them, we had sonograms done very early, at four or five weeks. With Susanna, due to some misunderstandings and scheduling problems, we did not get in for one until I was seven weeks along, and were severely reprimanded by that doctor for waiting too long. "You don't wait that long if you have a history of tubal pregnancy!"

Since we hadn't known that I was pregnant, I would say that my experience with a tubal pregnancy left me more emotionally traumatized by the physical trauma I went through than by any grieving for the loss of the pregnancy.

Since I had been so very alone through the final ordeal of it, it was hard for anyone else to imagine what I had faced. I feel a deep gratitude to God that He granted me the privilege of still being here to love and care for my family. I think the thread from life to death is very fragile.

Have faith and remember the sparrows,
God sees them and cares for them, too,
And you're far more precious than sparrows
So have faith, God is caring for you!

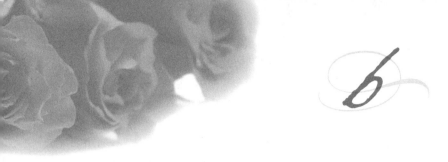

Joy Cometh in the Morning

—*Tessie M. Rutherford, McGrady, NC*

IN OCTOBER OF 2002, we had a son born to us. Since I do not have a cycle when I breast-feed till I'm feeding solids as well, I thought nothing of not having a cycle.

At the end of July 2003, I started having some problems. My side would hurt off and on. For a couple of days, it was really bad. I would sit doubled over in pain, and I asked my husband to pray extra hard.

Well, August began and my side was still bothering me somewhat, but not like it was earlier. With the other symptoms going on, I thought I was pregnant, but I did not have a pregnancy test at home and things worked out that I never took one. I had the feeling I was pregnant and something was very wrong.

On August 8, I felt awful. I was cramping and my side was really hurting again. These thoughts crossed my mind: either I was getting ready to start and had a cyst ready to burst, or I was getting ready to miscarry. Around 10:00 p.m. I went to the bathroom. I had a hard time getting there because of how badly my side hurt. When I got there, I thought I had started to miscarry. With such severe pain, I decided to take a pain pill. I explained to my husband what was going on, then took our son to bed, breast-fed him and fell into a very restless sleep.

Around 1:00 a.m. on the 9th, I woke up and knew I had to get to the bathroom before our son woke up to eat. (I still breast-fed at least once during the night.) I got another pain pill and went to feed the baby. After feeding him, I had to get to the bathroom. I woke up my husband, who put our very unhappy son in his playpen with some Cheerios to help calm him down. Then he came to check on me. I told him I thought I was probably miscarrying. After talking for a few minutes, he wondered if I was still using the bathroom. I explained that I was not, but I was bleeding so heavily that it sounded like I was using the bathroom.

He called the hospital and had them page my OB/GYN. When the doctor called back, he told us if I was hurting and bleeding that bad then something more was going on than just a miscarriage. If I was miscarrying, I should not have been experiencing as much pain and should not be bleeding so heavily. He recommended going to the hospital, with his office being closed the next day. We got off the phone, and my husband and I continued to talk and pray about what to do.

Later on, my husband told me I stopped answering him clearly and was leaning against the wall beside the toilet. I was quickly getting worse from the blood loss and pain. At this point, he called his brother, our next-door neighbor, to come help. He needed help to get me in the van and someone to get our three children, because something was very wrong.

I can remember them helping me to the van and telling our children I was going to the hospital, but everything would be fine. Our oldest daughter, who was eight at the time, knew we thought I was losing a baby and needed the doctor's help.

When I got to the hospital, they took us to admissions. As a nurse took my blood pressure, he started asking questions. He quickly realized how badly I was hurting and took me to an examination room to get some help, while my husband finished the paperwork. I remember the doctor telling me he had to have an ultrasound and blood work done before he could do anything.

They drew blood and sent me for an ultrasound. By now, I was hurting uncontrollably. The nurse could not get everything she needed, because she refused to put me through more pain. I remember when they started IV and got the pain to where I could handle it. The ER doctor came in and told us that he called my doctor. I don't remember if he told us that I had a pregnancy in my tube or if it was my doctor.

I do remember talking to my doctor. He sent me back for another ultrasound so he had a better idea of what to do. With the pain medications I was fine through the ultrasound. My doctor told us my tube was ruptured and I was bleeding uncontrollably. I needed surgery immediately. After calling our parents and pastor, I headed to pre-op. My husband and parents were there to pray with me as I was heading for surgery. Our pastor was there when I came in to the hospital room.

I had to stay overnight. I did not get to feed our son but once during my hospital stay. This was hard on me both physically and emotionally. I needed to be with him. When the doctor talked to us later, he told us he had to remove the tube because of all the damage. He also did a D&C.

That first week was very hard. I had to deal with losing the baby. I had no idea if I could have more children. I had to deal with the trauma of surgery and the fact that no one would give me any time alone. Because of the blood loss, I was very weak and had trouble getting from room to room, so the doctor's orders were not to leave me alone. I had to do everything under watchful eyes, whether it was eating, sleeping, resting, reading or praying. No matter what, someone was always there. I desperately wanted a few minutes to mourn and pray alone.

The next week I met a preacher's wife who had experienced a tubal pregnancy. Sharing with her helped me greatly. She said two things that helped. One was "to remember that God understands the pain because He had lost His Son." What a concept! God understands because He has been there. She also told me not to be afraid of the questions I had, but to go ahead and ask God, just to be willing to accept His answer, no matter what it was, even if I must wait indefinitely for the answer. Remember God knows our thoughts and our hearts, so go ahead and open up. Be honest with Him, talk with Him, and let Him do the healing.

Many others said many things. Some of these things hurt, like "Well, you have three others" and "You can have another baby." They didn't mean to hurt me, but they did not understand that others would never take the place of the one that is gone. Others said things that helped some. Some told me they had lost a baby and understood what I was going through. Some even admitted they had never been there, but knew it must hurt. Everyone offered prayer, which I am sure helped the most.

It took time to work through the emotional pain. My life's verse is Isaiah 26:3. "Thou wilt keep him in perfect peace, whose mind is stayed on thee: because he trusteth in thee." Another promise that I strongly believe is "Weeping may endure for a night, but joy cometh in the morning." That first time I had alone with God, He reminded me of these two verses. At that point, I started experiencing that peace that passes all understanding.

One month later, on September 9, we had a memorial service. Many friends and family did not understand, but they came anyway. Basically we had a funeral to publicly say we had a baby that passed on before us. This was a wonderful release to me. It was a chance to say good-bye for a little while and move forward.

Almost a year later, a friend miscarried. I was able to be there for her. It was another time of healing for me. Remembering what I had gone through and knowing some of what she would be experiencing, I was able to help her.

Now, 3 1/2 years later, I can say God does know what is best. In 2005, we learned we would have another baby. No, this child would not take the place of the one who passed on, but he is a new blessing from the Lord.

I had an emotional pregnancy. After learning that this pregnancy was not an ectopic, I was still afraid something would go wrong, and I would lose this baby too. This worry made me fight depression. I have since learned that this is a normal reaction, and my doctor was always checking to see how things were going physically, but mostly emotionally. He told me the signs to watch for and to be sure to seek help immediately if I thought I saw any warning signs that I was no longer able to fight the depression.

Due around Christmas 2005, we were pleasantly surprised when we arrived at the hospital on January 2, 2006, and learned that we were about to have the first baby in our county in the New Year.

If God blesses us with future children, I expect to go through some of the same feelings, but prayerfully things will go smoother the next time around.

I shall always remember and honor the baby we lost on August 8, 2003. I am still comforted by talking with others who have experienced a loss, and I expect I always shall. God bless and help each one of you who has had a similar loss.

There are many things in life
That we cannot understand,
But we must trust God's judgment
And be guided by His hand.
And all who have God's blessings
Can rest safely in His care,
For He promises "safe passage"
On the wings of faith and prayer.

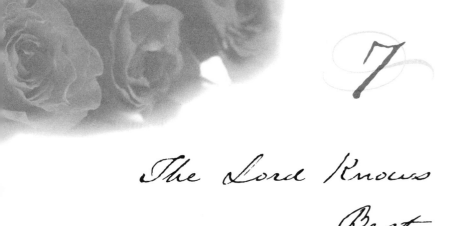

The Lord Knows Best

—Lerov & Rachel Hostetler, New Concord, OH

WE WERE MARRIED for a year and two months and had a three-month-old baby. When the baby was six weeks old, I had my first period. Two weeks later, I had my second one, but didn't think much about it. But then I started with severe pain in my side and down my left leg. It lasted for about an hour. But the ache just kind of stayed there. I used to get sick with my periods as a girl and thought maybe it would change after I had a child. Now this one was even worse.

My period lasted only three days, then it stopped for a few days and started again. The pain got worse at times. My mom thought it might be my gallbladder, as she had lots of trouble with hers. She gave me some pills to take.

A day or so later I was sewing and my legs hurt so much that I couldn't go on with my sewing. I went to talk with my mother, who lives on the same place we do.

My mom advised me to see our midwife. She thought I might be pregnant and it might be in my tubes. The thought of pregnancy had not even crossed my mind, and I didn't know of pregnancies being in the tube.

I decided that if I could get a neighbor to take me, I'd go, and if not, I'd just stay at home. Gas prices were high and it was almost 30 miles to the midwife. I couldn't get any of the neighbors to take me, but I had this uneasy feeling, so I decided I'd just get whoever is available. I called my husband at work, and he, too, advised me to go.

When we got to the midwife, I told her what's up. At first she thought I might have a tipped uterus. But then she noticed I was in pain all the while. She did a pregnancy test, and of course it showed positive. Then and there she decided it's probably in my tubes.

She asked to use the driver's cell phone to call the doctor. She worked in Coshocton. I was told to come in right away. It was after office hours till I got there. How I wished for my husband or Mom at my side! My driver tried to tell me she doesn't think I could be pregnant with a nursing three-month-old.

The doctor did another pregnancy test and an ultrasound. He said I'm four to six weeks pregnant, but he can't find anything. He told me to come back the next day if I'm still having pain.

The pain had been worsening all afternoon, and by that time I had to press my hand to my side to help ease the pain. When he noticed this, he told me I could go to the hospital right away if I preferred. There they could use a microscope to see what's wrong.

My head was spinning. What should I do? I didn't want to go to the hospital if nothing was wrong. Oh, if only Leroy were here with me! I tried to call Leory and Mom, but to no avail. In the end, the doctor advised me to go right away.

When I got to the emergency room, a long line of people were waiting. "Oh, no," I thought, "how much longer can I bear this pain?" But a Higher Hand was watching over me, as the people stepped back and let me go first. They must have noticed I was in pain. I didn't argue, but thanked them and gladly went ahead.

My driver went back home to get my husband and my mom. I got my paperwork done and the lady told me where to go. This was an unfamiliar surrounding for me and I was scared about riding the elevator by myself.

A rough-looking guy came over to me and offered to go with me. He must have heard me ask the nurse if I could wait till my husband comes. Anyway, I gladly went with him. It was only the two of us on the elevator, and I didn't even think of being afraid. He took me to the nurses' station and I thanked him. He never said anything.

I was taken to my room and given pain medication. All at once an itchy, red rash appeared on my arms, so they stopped giving it, and gave something else instead. It didn't take long until the pain left.

Leroy and Mom arrived just a little before I was taken to the operating room. How glad I was to see them! As I was wheeled into the operating room, the tears just flowed. I couldn't keep them back any longer.

The next thing I knew I was waking up in the recovery room, in great pain. They gave me all the pain medication they could.

I went home the next day, and sure was sore for a while! None of my tubes were ruptured, which we are very thankful for. The reason nothing showed up on the ultrasound was because too much blood was in the way.

The doctor said my tube could've burst at any time. He said it would probably happen again, one out of five times. It wasn't a very pleasant experience, but the Lord knows best.

It is now 1 1/2 years since my tubal and we didn't have any more children since. We hope we can have more some day. We have been blessed.

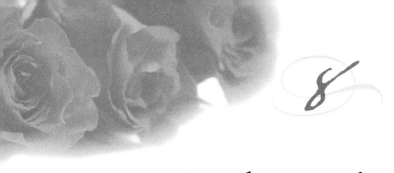

In God's Hands

—anonymous

IT WAS A warm summer day and I was weeding my flower bed. I had a queasy feeling, and each day after that a little morning sickness was felt. It was still a week before my period was due. The time came when a test was done, and sure enough, a pregnancy had begun.

We were happy, as our firstborn was nearing the age of two years. After a few weeks, the morning sickness lessened, till it was mild. I figured I'm slipping out of being sick this time, and never thought of losing the baby.

I started on housecleaning, but I couldn't keep on working like usual. I had to rest often and had a dull ache in my right side. I decided not to hurry with the work, but kept steadily on till Saturday. After supper I swept off the cement blocks like usual, all of a sudden wetness was felt. There was a gush of bright red blood, but it stopped again when I rested. That was the first time a feeling swept over me that this pregnancy might not last.

The next day, Sunday, we didn't trust going to church, as there was still a dull ache. And with the scare we'd had the evening before, we didn't know what was up. In the evening our next-door neighbors invited us over. We decided to go, as everything seemed okay again.

We were there only a little while till I felt myself becoming warmer and warmer. I decided to go back to our house, because I was really sweating. By the time I came to the kitchen, I had a sharp pain and a bright red gush of blood.

In the meantime, when I didn't show up again at the neighbors, my husband came to check up on me and found me on the floor in sharp pain. We didn't know what we should do, till my dear husband said he's going to call the midwife. She asked us to go straight to the hospital, as it might be appendicitis or a tubal pregnancy.

The neighbor took us in to the hospital, and by the time we got there, the pain was only a dull ache. Everyone was busy in the hospital that evening and we waited about two hours before they checked me out. A tubal pregnancy was found.

Two o'clock in the morning surgery was done. They told us we were fortunate because it would have burst that morning yet. What saved the tube from bursting was a leak where blood leaked out, giving some relief. The only part of the tube that was lost was where the baby had been attached. We were told it was a nice little one, and because of the size, they guessed it to be eight or nine weeks along. We don't know if this tube is active or not. The doctor said it just depends if the tube has scar tissue.

After that disappointment, recovery began. That first week after coming home from the hospital, I had trouble sleeping, until the hormones straightened out. After that I recovered quickly.

My arms felt empty and I grieved a little. A big help to me was a letter the hospital sent out. They sent a letter of sympathy, along with what all you may feel after a tubal pregnancy or miscarriage. It said you're a very normal person to have these feelings. That was a big comfort to me.

We just didn't know if we would have more children or not. We tried to leave it all in God's hands. We were still young and our child-bearing age wasn't over yet. It helped a lot to keep myself occupied, especially doing things for other people.

Guess what! Seven months later we were overjoyed that I was pregnant again. But fear filled our hearts, when at five weeks, I had a lot of pain in my other tube. We went to the hospital for an ultrasound, but nothing was found to be wrong. The pain kept on till about eight weeks, when it just disappeared. Otherwise it was a healthy pregnancy, and in the end we were blessed with our first girl!

Two years later we were blessed with another boy, and two and a half years after that, we had our third boy. With each pregnancy after the tubal, there was much pain in my tubes until I was about eight weeks along. We didn't go for an ultrasound with the last two pregnancies. We just watched for unusual signs.

I am again about three months along. This time there was almost no pain in my tubes, but I had more severe morning sickness than I had with all the other pregnancies. We are hoping this will also be a full-term baby. We have so many blessings to be thankful for.

An Eastern Shepherd

An Eastern shepherd led his sheep
Toward a river's brink,
But when they saw the stream was broad
Their hearts with fear did shrink;
And though the shepherd went across
In view of all the sheep,
They did not dare to follow him
And ford the waters deep.

And so he took a little lamb
Right from its mother's side,
He clasped it in his shelt'ring arm,
And with it crossed the tide.
The mother, missing what she loved,
Was eager now to gain
The distant shore, that she might find
Her precious lamb again.

She quickly made her way across,
And soon the stream she passed;
And other sheep soon followed her,
'Til all had crossed at last.
She found the lamb which she had lost,
Within the shepherd's care;
And he had used her little one,
In leading many there.

Oh, Mother, has your little lamb
Been carried on before?
The Shepherd wants to have you, too,
Upon the farther shore.
And so He clasped your treasured one
Unto His sheltering breast,
That you might come and seek it there,
And find in Him your rest.

In days to come it may be we shall see
Just why was sent this bitter test;
'Til then, we can but bow our head in tears,
And say, "God knoweth best."

—*Author Unknown*

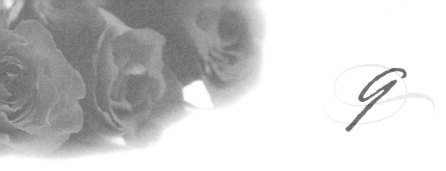

My Grace Is Sufficient

—Willis & Becky Coblentz, Millersburg, OH

"WHAT TIME I am afraid, I will trust in thee" (Psalm 56:3).

It happened on a Saturday morning. I climbed out of bed with severe pain in my abdomen. When my husband came in from doing chores, I was lying on my stomach on the bathroom floor. Thinking it might be appendicitis, he helped me up on the bed and got me to hang over the side. That didn't feel good at all, and didn't help matters any. The pain was going up into my chest and affecting my breathing.

By this time our five-year-old was awake. I tried to be brave and hide the tremendous pain, but I just couldn't. All I could think was, "Get me to the emergency room!"

My husband's sister arrived to stay with our three children: Sierra, 5, Benjamin, 3, and Mahalah, 2. When we arrived at the hospital they had me lie on a bed. The doctor pushed around on my belly, asking where I felt the pain. It hurt wherever he pushed!

I had to go to the bathroom to get a urine sample, but there I passed out. I remember thinking, "Ahh, this sure feels good!"

Meanwhile they had done a blood test, which revealed that I was pregnant. What a surprise!

Now they rushed about. They took an ultrasound, which showed a pregnancy in the tube. It had burst and quite a bit of blood was gushing out. In a matter of minutes, they were pushing me through the doors of the operating room. Then I was put to sleep. (That was nice!)

One third of my tube was removed. If necessary, he can fix that one up and it can still be used.

Having had three C-sections prior to this, I was familiar with surgeries. This time it was different. I didn't have the joy of a precious, sweet-smelling baby to help ease the pain. "My grace is sufficient for thee..." I remember I felt like bursting into tears when my mom came in to see me.

I stayed at the hospital for two days. When you get cut open during surgery, some air gets in there, and oh! what pain! Coming home on Monday, April 3, 2006, things looked quite overwhelming to me. "My grace is sufficient for thee, for my strength is made perfect in weakness." This verse came to my mind again. God is good—He is with us in all things.

You really feel the need for others when you're in this state. My husband would get up during the night and make grape juice eggnog for me. Midwife Freida Miller told me to take this to help regain my strength. (Beat two raw eggs then fill the glass with grape juice.) This really helped. I wasn't sure I could get it down, but it really didn't taste too bad. Even our children liked it!

My nieces came to help us out. Family stopped in with cookies, flowers and all kinds of goodies. Our church families brought in meals. What a blessing to have such caring people around us. We are blessed—may we ever be thankful!

Three weeks into recovery, my husband was backing up

a tractor and trailer. Our three-year-old son was sleeping behind the wheel, where Dad didn't notice him. The trailer wheels went across the top part of his leg and lower abdomen. We rushed him into the emergency room. He had a broken femur bone and bruised liver. After being in the hospital for three days, he had to be in a body cast for six weeks.

"But, Lord, I'm not supposed to do any lifting. How will I take care of him?" I wondered. "My grace is sufficient for thee..." once again!

"God is good and everything he does is good" (Psalm 119:68). Do we believe this? He brings these things into our lives, because He loves us, "that we might be partakers in his holiness" (Hebrews 12:10).

> I care not today what tomorrow may bring,
> If shadow or sunshine or rain,
> The Lord I know ruleth over everything
> And all of my worry is vain.

A TEAR FROM MY HEART

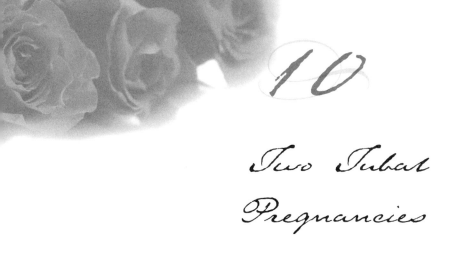

10

Two Tubal Pregnancies

—Junior & Ellen Keim, Topeka, IN

IT WAS DECEMBER of 2005. I was making supper and baking cookies. I was two weeks late with my period, but I thought nothing of it. Suddenly I had sharp pains in my right lower abdomen. I put supper on the table and went to the bathroom, but that didn't help. So I sat at the table bent over. By the time supper was over, the pain had let up, so I did dishes, etc.

For a week I would get these sudden sharp pains, but they wouldn't last very long. Then I began spotting, and I figured that will be the end of it. But it wasn't.

On Friday, December 23, we went to the doctor. He guessed that I only had a hard period. But he advised us to do an ultrasound the next morning to make sure. There they found a tubal pregnancy. I had surgery that afternoon yet. The doctor just cut the tube, took the pregnancy out and sewed the tube back together. He advised me not to get pregnant for three months.

In May and June I had very hard periods. Then in July we were camping out behind our house beside the pond. We came to our own beds for the night. Thursday evening Darryl (almost 5) was sleeping, so I carried him up to the house. The next evening (the 7th) I carried Mary Alice (2) up to her bed. I had to stop when I was partways up, as my back was so sore. After I'd put Mary Alice to bed, I had a sudden sharp pain in my stomach again, but I figured it will get better again. Surely it was not a tubal again. But I did not get much sleep that night, as I was in such pain.

Saturday was the last day for the campers. After breakfast they wanted to pack up and leave, so I wanted to eat breakfast with them too. But I couldn't stand sitting in a chair, so I went back to my bed.

My husband went to town and got a pregnancy test kit, which showed positive. He called the doctor, who asked us to go to the hospital for an ultrasound. I had not even known I was pregnant. But with the blood tests and ultrasound, they said I am indeed pregnant, but the baby isn't living anymore. They did a D&C and we went home again.

At 4:00 the next morning when I went to the bathroom, I started sweating and had a roaring sound in my ears. I asked my husband to help me back to bed. It was Sunday morning and my husband was planning to attend church. Sister Dorene was going to bring the children home and stay with me till he returned.

At 8:00 my husband helped me to the bathroom, but I just couldn't walk anymore, so I went back to bed. Every time I moved around in bed I got hot and sweaty, so I tried to hold as still as possible.

When my husband came home from church, he put Mary Alice to bed, and Devon (3) fell asleep beside me. Then my husband and Dorene helped me go to the bathroom again. Before we got there, I passed out. So he called the doctor, who said, "Bring her in." He came back into the house, took one look at me, then went out and called the ambulance.

When we got to the hospital, the doctor pushed on my stomach three times. "I think you are bleeding internally," he announced. He called the surgery team in, which took another hour. I was in severe pain, as it was pushing into my chest, around my sides into my back. I was gasping for breath and whenever I stopped, they talked to me to keep me conscious. The last I remember was when they rolled me into the operating room.

I woke up very weak and thirsty. The doctor had dipped four pints of blood out and the rest had to be absorbed by my body. Besides the one in the uterus, I also had a pregnancy in the same tube it happened in before. I also had a cyst on my ovary that was bleeding slowly. So they took out my right ovary and tube.

I was given four units of blood. My blood count was at seven when I went home. We received a lot of help, mail and visitors, which helped a lot.

I am now pregnant again and due in May. My body wasn't quite recovered yet, but we hope everything will turn out okay this time.

> The Lord is my strength and my song, and he has become my salvation.
> Exodus 15:2

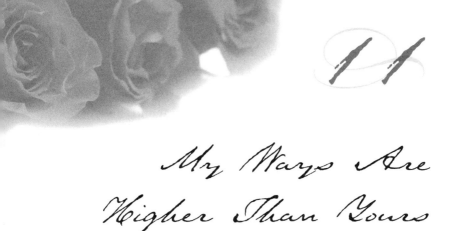

My Ways Are Higher Than Yours

—Tara L. Eby, Cabins, WV

IN JANUARY 1998, I experienced a tubal pregnancy. We had a ten-month-old baby and I had never had my regular cycle yet, so I didn't even know I was pregnant. I spotted off and on and had discomfort in my abdomen, but I never once thought of a tubal pregnancy.

One evening I was giving our little son a bath and chatting with my husband when the pain just kept getting worse. My husband told me to take Tylenol and lie down and he would finish bathing our son.

When my husband saw me rolling back and forth on our bed and moaning and groaning, he called the doctor. Right away the doctor thought it sounded like a tubal pregnancy, and wanted us to go to the emergency room immediately. It was 8:30 in the evening.

The first thing they did in the hospital was take a pregnancy test. It came back positive. Next they took a sonogram and could not find the baby. They could see blood and fluid around my uterus. So around midnight, they did surgery and found my right fallopian tube partially ruptured.

I remember waking up and thinking, "At least the pain will be gone now." But I was wrong. I ended up getting bladder infection after the surgery, and it wasn't until four weeks later that I started feeling better.

I had been nursing our son up to this point and thought it would be over now. But a few days after the surgery, I was able to continue nursing.

I cried a lot! I had been praying for another little one; and to realize God had answered my prayer only to take him back to Him, brought me joy and grief at the same time.

Songs and hymns really brought comfort to my broken heart. Even though I didn't feel like singing, listening to tapes brought healing. I knew God's ways were best and He was in control, and that brought peace to my soul.

Yet I struggled with fear when I'd think about how I had only one tube now and what if my next pregnancy was also a tubal pregnancy. It was nine months before I conceived again. These were probably one of the longest and hardest nine months! I had to keep committing my future, my desires, my womb, my everything to the Lord. Everything I have is from God. Everything He gives me is for His glory. Looking back, I wouldn't want to trade those months for anything! They were a time of crying to the Lord and feeling His tender arms carrying me through. Praise His name!

There was an article I read shortly after my tubal pregnancy that was a blessing to me. It told about a mother who had a two-year-old son who died 24 hours after coming down with a fever. Fourteen years later the same mother had the pain of a rebellious son. She admits it was her own selfish grief and bitterness. It stole her joy, leaving her without a smile to nurture her living son. She said, "It would have been easier to have also lost this one to death as a baby than to see what has become of him now."

That spoke to me. I did not want to become bitter. I wanted to be the mother God wanted me to be for the child I did have. Someday I will see our little one in Heaven.

Now nine years later, God has blessed us with two more boys and two girls. We also experienced a molar pregnancy between our two girls. "For my thoughts are not your thoughts, neither are your ways my ways, saith the Lord. For as the heavens are higher than the earth, so are my ways higher than your ways, and my thoughts than your thoughts" (Isaiah 55:8 & 9).

Life is a mixture
of sunshine and rain,
Teardrops and laughter,
pleasure and pain.
We can't have all bright days,
but one thing is true:
No cloud is so dark
that the sun can't shine through.

I Need You, Lord

We know God's way is best,
But still we wonder, "Why?"
We wanted you, oh precious one,
Why did you have to die?

Oh, give us hearts that sweetly say,
"Lord, may Thy will be done.
You gave, and now you took away
This darling little one."

Lord, take away the bitterness,
The sadness and the strife,
Fill, Thou, the emptiness that's left
Within our heart and life.

Only with Thee can we bear
The hurt and loneliness
Of empty arms and shattered dreams,
The sorrow and the stress.

—*Author Unknown*

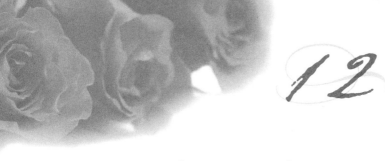

12

Just One More

—*anonymous*

ONE LOVELY FRIDAY morning in September I got up as usual. I sat on the sofa to put on my shoes. As I bent down there was an awful stabbing pain in the area of my rectum. My first thoughts were severe gas pains, yet I had never experienced anything like it before.

It wouldn't let up, so I went to the bathroom, thinking it may get better. No relief. So I finally took Tylenol to help bear the pain. I had to help the school girls get ready to leave on time. After half an hour or so, I felt fine again and dismissed the whole thing from my mind.

Saturday morning the same thing happened again, only worse. But after awhile everything was all right again. This began to puzzle me. Then a slight spotting appeared for a while. I remember telling my husband I wonder if it could be a tubal pregnancy. Yet I thought those are usually more severe and life-threatening. Oh well, I'm all right yet.

Later in the day the pain came back again, with heavier spotting. Whatever could be the matter? I had my period only two weeks before. The midwife was not at home that weekend and I did not feel this urgent enough to contact her.

Sunday morning came and we all went to church. All was fine until we were ready to leave for home. The pain came again with continuous heavy spotting. It was pure torture to drive home from church. Every jolt of the wheels sent pain that felt like a knife turning in my rectal area. After arriving at home we decided it's time I take it easy and prop up my feet.

On Monday the midwife told me she expects I have an infection in my tube. So on Tuesday I made a doctor appointment. The doctor felt I have a cyst on the ovary and need to watch what I do for awhile. But he still wanted me to get a blood test taken at the hospital just to check my hormone level. I was so glad when that half hour ride home was over.

Ten minutes after arriving at home, the phone rang. "Your hormone count is up, so I need to do an ultrasound. Come to my office right away."

So off to the doctor we went again. The ultrasound showed a dark spot on my tube and a large dark area of pooled blood in the abdominal cavity. I was admitted to the hospital to be operated on a couple hours later.

The doctor was very concerned about how I feel, but wanted to wait until after his office hours to operate if possible. An hour after surgery I was waking up. I had a small opening where they had entered with the camera. But there was too much blood, so they made a larger incision to be able to see.

The pain, they told me, was caused by bleeding into tissues where it doesn't belong. The one doctor told me, "You are lucky. We get them in here bleeding like a faucet turned open. We can hardly work fast enough."

I was six or seven weeks pregnant, even though my period was only two weeks before. I was told that pregnancy in a tube does not give off enough hormones to shut down the cycle.

The place where the tube had ruptured only caused it to bleed by spurts. The doctor just took out the baby and left the tube, saying it often works all right. They cleaned out a pint of blood as well. I was allowed to go home and continue nursing our six-month-old baby.

Life continued and I was not really concerned. The doctor had told me to keep a home pregnancy kit on hand. As soon as I suspect I am pregnant and it shows positive, I need to come to his office for an ultrasound.

In January, four months later, on a Sunday afternoon I was pulling the girls on a sled. I felt just a slight hint of pain again, but I tried to ignore it.

On Monday I did the laundry. Now I could no longer ignore the pain, as it was more severe. Even though my period was only two weeks before, I used the test kit. It showed positive. I could have cried on the spot, for we knew the answer.

A call to the doctor brought an appointment the next day with the same results. Another surgery. Another big incision. This time it was only trickling, but he removed the tube.

> Faith is a **Fantastic Adventure In** **Trusting Him.**

There was too much scar tissue and 100% chance for another tubal. This time around brought an abrupt end to the nursing of our now ten-month-old baby.

Now I was more concerned. I really wished for just one more. Every month was an up and down seesaw. Finally, eleven months later, a few days after my period was due, I started to feel pressure on the side where I still had a tube.

The test kit showed positive, so off for another ultrasound. Again a dark spot showed on the tube and I had an elevated hormone count. The following day I was admitted on observation.

Some ladies get badly upset stomachs from this shot, but I didn't. A few days later I was to get another blood test done. The hormone count was even higher, so I was given another shot. I was given a number of different warning signs, and if any showed up, I should go to the ER immediately. My, how stressful!

Twenty-four hours later my pain got pretty bad, so we headed for the hospital. Now the ultrasound showed two dark spots—one in the uterus and one in the tube. The doctor said if there are two babies we'll be in trouble.

The decision was made to operate, remove the tube and do a D&C to avoid hemorrhaging. I had to wait several hours until the OR was empty.

Many thoughts ran through my mind. Our baby was not quite two years old. How we had hoped for just one more! Especially after having parted with a newborn a little over three years before and later having another healthy one.

I looked out the window, longing to be anywhere else but on the hospital bed, all prepared for surgery. "Oh, for wings like a dove, to fly away..." Yet at the same time it was a relief to be through with the stress of living under such life-threatening conditions.

The doctor remarked how the tube did not look like tubal pregnancies often do. He sent that and the D&C to the lab.

Two weeks later I was back for another checkup. The lab results showed a pregnancy in the uterus and a chronic infection in the tube. There were pockets of fluid causing the pressure and the dark spots on the ultrasound. He figured the pregnancy would have ended up as a miscarriage and the tube would never have functioned again.

Just like that, our family was complete, with six girls living. Health was granted and life continues. The healing of the emotions took much longer than the physical healing.

A note from the husband: Although we will always wonder if that last pregnancy would have worked out, there are no guilt feelings. The stress of that pregnancy was tremendous on our nerves. We were warned to be at the emergency room in less than one hour if symptoms appear. They said even that is too long, but they realized it is the best we can do. The relief of rescuing my wife from under that dark cloud greatly overrides any possible guilt feeling. I know both the doctor and we did the best we knew under the circumstances. At any rate, we realize now that living without fear is a wonderful feeling!

Oft upon the rock I tremble,
Faint of heart and weak of knee,
But the solid Rock of Ages
Never trembles under me.

Prayer of the Afflicted

My God, my God,
I call to Thee.
Do Thou make haste
To answer me.
Out of the depths
Of deep despair
My soul doth groan—
Dost Thou yet care?

Where art Thou, God?
I grope to find
Thy outstretched Hand,
So firm and kind.
I grope and feel
No tender touch.
Oh, Father, hear!
I need so much.

Tears overflow
My swollen eye;
I think they never
Will run dry.
I cannot see
For tears and pain.
How can such loss
Work Heaven's gain?

And yet I know
That Thou art strong,
And Thou wilt not
Leave me too long.
To sink beneath
This bleak despair,
But soon again
I'll feel Thy care.

When my emotions'
Highest tide,
Shall crest at last
And then subside,
I yet shall feel
Beneath my feet,
Salvation's Rock,
So strong and sweet.

I yet shall find
That Thou wast near,
Although Thy voice
I could not hear.
Though storm winds howl
And I must grieve,
I still shall pray
And still believe.

—L.B

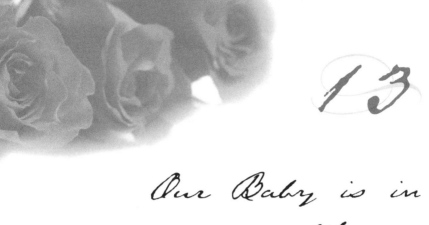

13

Our Baby is in Heaven

—anonymous

IT WAS A hot, dry summer in July 2006. But all that didn't seem to matter, for we had just discovered that we were expecting a baby! What happiness there was, for this was our first, and it seemed we had waited for a long time.

We couldn't keep such wonderful news to ourselves very long. We soon shared it with our immediate families. What excitement! This would be the first grandchild on both sides. My mother and mother-in-law gave me some dos and don'ts. "Now take your vitamins. Drink lots of water. Take it a little easy, and don't lift too heavy."

We called the doctor's office to set up our first appointment. It was scheduled for the tenth week of my pregnancy. The nurse told me that if I had any problems before then, I was to call and they would see me right away. I was in the sixth week, so another month seemed far away.

I was only a little sick, but *so* tired all the time. All that was normal, though, and I didn't give it any thought that something could go wrong. Shortly afterward I started with pain in my lower abdomen. It just appeared occasionally. My husband

and I talked it over and decided it just goes with pregnancy.

Gradually the pains became worse. It was really sharp in my right side, but then it would slowly taper off and I would be fine again. I didn't think too much about it. I wasn't spotting like I had earlier.

One evening when we were washing dishes, the pain flew into my side again. I grabbed onto the sink, as I thought I was going to pass out. My husband helped me to the couch. I just lay there, wondering what could be wrong. *Do I have appendicitis? Is it a tubal pregnancy? No, these are pretty rare.* I had ovarian cysts before, but this felt a little different. Again the pain left, so I assumed I was okay.

It was Sunday, the beginning of the eighth week, and we were at my parents for dinner. Everything seemed fine until

> He does not lead me year by year
> Nor even day by day,
> But step by step my path unfolds—
> My Lord directs my way.

that afternoon when I once again had a "pain attack." This time it was worse than ever, and altogether different. Instead of sharp pain, I had abdominal pressure. I thought it felt like I hadn't gone to the bathroom in weeks! I felt nauseous, and so weak for a while that I thought I was going to die.

Mom wanted me to go to the emergency room, because all the doctors' offices were closed. But I didn't want to. I wasn't spotting, and besides, I disliked hospitals.

An hour later the pain was gone. I was still tender and sore, but otherwise I felt just fine. That evening when we got home my husband made me promise I would call the doctor the next morning and tell them what was going on. I should also get an appointment as soon as possible.

Monday morning I called the doctor and told the nurse about the happenings over the weekend, but that I was fine now. She told me that sometimes the baby rearranges things and causes discomfort. But I should call if anything changes. That evening I had a little spotting, but my pregnancy book said some people do spot a little, so I wasn't too worried.

Tuesday morning my doctor called and was quite worried. The nurse had told her what was going on. "I really want you to come in today if you can," she said. So I quickly got a driver and went to her office. For the first time, I was shaken up.

Everything went well, and we discovered my due date is on my mother's birthday! But no ultrasound could be done until the next day. I really didn't want to go again, so I asked them if I really had to. "Yes, you should, just to make sure it's not a tubal pregnancy or something else going wrong." Concerned about the tubal pregnancy, I inquired, "Do you really feel that it might be that?" The nurse said she didn't think so, as at 49 days I would be in constant, unbearable pain.

My husband and I were concerned about this. We prayed about it, and asked both sets of parents to pray for us. Knowing everything was in Higher Hands, we could both rest better.

The next morning I left for the doctor's office once again. My husband thought he should take off from work and accompany me. But I knew he needed to work, as this was going to cost quite a sum of money. I assured him that I would be just fine.

In the ultrasound room, I didn't like what I saw. I couldn't read the ultrasound screen like the experts can, but I could read the technician's face clearly. Snappily she asked when my last period was and all the rest. Then she said, " I just don't see anything! I have to get your doctor!" With that, she left.

I wondered, *Okay, and what was that supposed to mean? Am I not even pregnant?* I was *so* glad to see my doctor come in just then, as she is a super nice person and *so* caring. She carefully explained everything. It could be one of two things. Either I wasn't as far along as I'd thought, or it was a tubal pregnancy.

I was sent to the hospital next door to have blood work done to check my HCG level. This would tell her exactly how far along I was. Then she told me to go home and pray and think positive. There was no sense in worrying until we knew. She said she'd call in the morning as soon as she got the results. If I had any serious bleeding or more pain attacks, I was to go straight to the hospital.

How was I to break this news to my husband? Could they just transplant the baby into my uterus? Questions and more questions whirled through my head when I got home. Thankfully, our neighbors had gone on a trip and I had offered to baby-sit their three-year-old. That kept my mind occupied till my husband arrived.

The doctor called the next morning with the results. I'd have to go back to the hospital the following morning to get more blood work done. Then I'd have to come to her office. If the HCG levels had doubled, she would know everything is fine, for I would just not be as far along as I had thought. Whew! I felt so much better. Maybe everything would be all right.

I explained to the little boy I was baby-sitting that we would be going away the next day. If he thinks he can be a good boy, he can go along. Of course, he thought he could. We packed some books, toys and coloring books. My youngest sister wanted to go along and watch him for me. My mother also offered to go along. I was relieved, as she understood all the hospital terms and all that complicated stuff. Again, my husband thought he should go, but we decided it would be all right if he goes to work. I could call him at work if I received any bad news. The pain had subsided, but I was spotting again.

Friday, August 4, 2006—a day we would never forget. I was one day close to eight weeks. I packed up the little boy, again breathing a thankful prayer that I had him to keep me occupied, besides my sister and my mother.

We headed to the hospital for blood work. One nurse exclaimed, "Girl, what have you done?" I had black and blue bruises all over my arms. My veins like to "jump" from needles. Often it takes the second nurse till they get the blood taken. This time they found a vein on the back of my hand that wasn't bruised, or didn't "jump." We then went to the hospital cafeteria for breakfast before heading back to my doctor's office.

My doctor took me in for another ultrasound and said the results of the HCG should be back any minute. Just then her pager went off and she left to check the results. When she returned she looked at the ultrasound and the results once more.

I can still hear her words as if she'd said them just yesterday. "Looking at your HCG levels and the ultrasound, I am so sorry, but this is a tubal pregnancy." She stepped out the door, and I just held on to my mom and cried.

"Why? Dear Lord, why? I wanted this baby so much..."

All too soon the doctor came back. I could see she had been crying too. She quietly explained everything that was to happen, and answered all my questions. I would be going in for surgery immediately, as my tube could rupture at any time, and then we would have more problems.

She showed me to the phone. With a heavy heart, I called

my husband. This wasn't what I preferred telling him on the phone, but I got it choked out. He told me to hang in there; he'd come right away. He was working about an hour's drive away, but fortunately a driver was there to bring him to the hospital.

Everything was happening so fast. My mind just went numb. In just a short while that beating heart inside me would be gone. I did not want to go for surgery. They were going to kill my baby. I decided to refuse going for surgery until my husband arrived. All these thoughts were whirling around in my head. I knew the surgery had to be done, and I tried to keep a smile on my face.

We went slowly to the hospital, where I checked in and they said they'd call my number. In the waiting room I tried to make light of everything. I hugged and talked to the little boy. I asked him if he's having fun playing toys with my sister. "Yes, but I'm about tired of them. Can we go home soon?" he asked. I would have loved to grab him and run home. My mom said if he gets too bored, she would send him and my sister home.

When will my husband get here? Does he know where the hospital is? I can't go for surgery without seeing him first!

"Number 6," the nurse called. Gulp—*that's my number.* Slowly I walked up to the desk. I told her I can't go in yet as my husband isn't here. She said it takes a long time to get everything ready, and they won't put me to sleep before he comes.

We filled out all kinds of paperwork, then I was put into a small, curtained room. The nurse came in and gave me this hideous gown to put on, that opened down the back. I waited awhile, because I didn't want to greet my husband in that ugly thing! The nurse returned and wondered if I need help to put the gown on. I was embarrassed about being worried over such a minor issue. My husband would not care what I was wearing. So I put it on, then they started IV. Now I really looked scary.

Just then my husband arrived. He looked really pale, but I sensed he was being strong for my sake. After talking things over with my husband, I felt so much better.

The doctor I'd had all along was going to do my surgery. I was so glad, as I knew and trusted her. She came and explained everything again to my husband.

"They are going to do this the laser method," she explained. "I am going to put a laparoscope into your belly button and make two small incisions. One will be an inch and the other half an inch." She also assured us she would try to save my tube, but if she sees it would cause too much scarring, she would remove it.

"I will try my best to save the tube," she promised. She would slit the tube, take the baby out, and it would heal back together. But too much scar tissue would just cause another tubal pregnancy.

The anesthesia doctor came in to talk with us, and I remembered Mom had wanted to talk with him. When my mom came and told him of a distant cousin of mine that had died from anesthesia, he almost laughed at her.

He replied that malignant hyperthermia susceptible (being allergic to certain anesthesia drugs) is extremely rare. And this being only a distant cousin, I should be fine. I never had anesthesia before, and my mother kept insisting they take all precautions. He then agreed to do everything as though I had hyperthermia. They would use different drugs, but I would still be in an unknowing sleep.

By now I admit I was terrified about having surgery. But I didn't let anyone know. Before being wheeled down the long hall, I got a quick kiss from my husband. I was taken into a cold room, praying all the while.

When I came back to my senses, I was wide awake. The clock told me I was in surgery one hour and forty-five minutes longer than they had said it would take. I asked the nurse for my family, but was told I'm in recovery and they can't come in here.

"Please tell them I'm okay," I urged. I imagined how terrible the wait must have been. "Can I talk to my doctor?" I asked. The nurse told me I couldn't until I was awake.

I felt like saying, "Excuse me. I happen to be very awake and I want to know what happened." But I kept silent. It felt as though everything in my entire middle section had been rearranged. It hurt to cough, but the nurse said I have to cough to get the fluid off my lungs.

My doctor came in and said she couldn't save my tube. The other one is still in good condition and she could see no reason why I can't have more children.

At that point, I didn't know how I felt about everything. I was still numb, but I thanked her over and over. I did not want to go through this again.

She also told me I am very lucky, as I do have hyperthermia. Even with every precaution taken, my blood pressure went dangerously high, and my heart rate faltered. If Mom had not warned them, I might have never made it through surgery.

I was taken to my room where I could finally see my husband. My mother, sister and a restless boy came in to visit before they left for home. We made arrangements for the little guy to go to his aunt and uncle.

It was now early evening, and the doctor said I'd have to stay for the night. We both tried to get some sleep. I was released the next morning with strict orders.

The following days and weeks were hard, both emotionally and physically. I was very thankful for the cards, letters, visitors and meals that were sent in by friends and family. I received a beautiful poem that was so healing to me:

Heaven's Nursery

In Heaven there must surely be
A special place, a nursery,
Where "little spirits" not fully grown
Go to live in their Heavenly home.

The angels must attend with love,
Tiny spirits on wings of doves,
The choir of angels must sing lullabies,
Maybe quieten their tiny cries.

The Father must come by each day
To cuddle and play in a special way,
These tiny spirits left earth too soon,
Little ones called Home from the womb.

These sparks of life did not perish
But came to the Father's love to cherish,
To grow and be taught in His own arms,
Safely away from all earthy harm.

The Comforter was sent to earth at once
To the parents who lost their little one.
Their hearts so ache, their arms feel empty,
The question "why" seems so tempting.

Then all at once in the midst of tears
There comes a peace that stills the fears,
The parents share the Father's own need
To hold their tiny spirit being.

They relinquish their own desperate hold
And release their baby to the Father's fold,
Then comes an angel to whisper the truth
Of a nursery in Heaven bearing rich fruit.

Of tiny spirits chosen to worship the Father,
A place that couldn't be filled by another,
Called to be spared from the struggles of earth,
Chosen to be one of Heaven's births.

So Father, whisper words of life from me
To our unborn "life" in Your nursery.
—Rebekah Milne

Time eases pain and hurt. We don't have our baby we so
longed for, but we have part of our family awaiting us on the
other shore.

Looking back, I feel truly blessed. My tube hadn't ruptured,
and there is still hope for children some day. We are so thankful
my mother was with us to warn the doctor of a possible
reaction. I know I would never have thought of telling them.

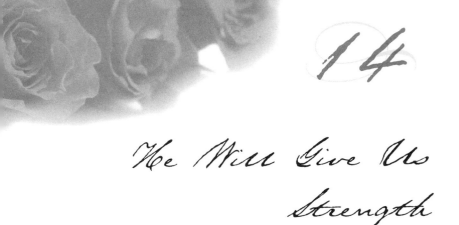

14

He Will Give Us Strength

—*Harvey & Barbara Byler, Dover, DE*

I'M PREGNANT AGAIN! Oh, what joy! It's my second pregnancy. With my first pregnancy I miscarried, and now, almost three years later, we are very happy that I am pregnant again.

I had so much pain at first that I was afraid something's wrong. So I went in to see my OB-GYN doctor right away, and they had me do blood work, to see if my levels would go up.

What a big disappointment when my levels did not go up! I was around seven weeks pregnant. An ultrasound was done, but nothing showed in my uterus. Another pregnancy test was done, which showed I'm still pregnant.

The doctor's next option was to do a D&C, which was a new experience for me. I thought that was very painful, but I experienced a lot more pain later.

After my D&C I was almost beside myself. I called my friend that had brought me in, and asked her to come and be with me, as my husband wasn't there to lean on. She helped me decide to get the shot, which would dissolve my tubal pregnancy. Her presence was a big comfort to me.

We had to go to the hospital for the shot. Here we met my mother-in-law, as her mom was also a patient. My mother-in-law stayed with me while my friend went to get my husband. Just being with my mother-in-law and talking about it helped me get control of myself. But I was glad to see my husband arrive, too.

We had to wait about five hours till I finally got my shot and got to go home. We picked up my sister on the way home to help out a few days.

The next day I helped my sister a little, and walked to the phone and to my brother's house, never realizing that I shouldn't. That night it started...oh, what pain! I guess I learned the hard way.

My husband called the doctor the next morning, as I could hardly bear the pain anymore. But the doctor told us this is normal. The following two weeks I had to be really careful or I had indescribable pain.

One day when I felt really down, I received a card with these words: "With God every day is a day to hope for the very best, to believe our prayers are being heard, to believe good news is on its way, and that anything can happen between yesterday and tomorrow." It was the only card I received, and to me it was the best medicine.

Two years later I had another miscarriage. If it is the Lord's will and everything goes fine, we should be blessed with our first baby in about eight weeks.

"Whenever God gives us a cross to bear, it is a promise that He will also give us strength."

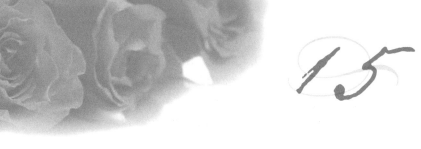

Great Is Our Lord

—Anna Mary Swartz, Petersburg, WV

IT WAS SIX weeks after our marriage over thirty years ago that I began to get more and more uncomfortable in the lower abdomen. Some days earlier, I had a general physical. The doctor noticed some tenderness in my abdomen. He thought it might be gas, and recommended paregoric. He later said that the thought of a tubal had crossed his mind, but he didn't think we'd been married long enough.

I didn't agree with his diagnosis and did nothing about it at that point. I had more and more pain. Some days later the tube ruptured and I lost much blood into the abdomen and had emergency surgery that evening. I soon felt much better and the Lord healed me rapidly and well.

Emotionally I did well too, as we were so new in our marriage. I felt it just might and possibly will go better, so I was okay.

Eleven months later I gave birth to our first child. So then the thoughts for sure were that things now were okay.

About fifteen months after the birth of our child, I had pain like the first time, so I didn't delay seeking help. I went to my gynecologist and he scheduled me for exploratory surgery the next day. I had a ruptured tube, a ruptured cyst and a ruptured ovary. Again the Lord was merciful and healed me quickly.

As far as my emotions, my husband and I wanted the Lord's will and it didn't bother me so much then as when I got quite a bit older and others were having children. I had prayed much and often, and felt this was the Lord's will for us and just went on with life, but not without disappointments time and again.

Having experienced two tubal pregnancies, I asked my gynecologist about it happening again. I didn't desire that of course. He said it would not happen again. I'm not sure why. Perhaps because of the extent of my surgeries.

What a *tremendous* help my husband was over the years, helping me again and again to look to God who in His wisdom does not make any mistakes.

With the very first experience, I don't know why I didn't seek the advice of a second doctor when I felt the diagnosis was incorrect. One wants to have confidence in the doctor, so I left it there.

With the second tubal, I don't really know if I knew I was having problems or thought I was expecting, so it came as a surprise. But again we must go with God in His wisdom and leave it there, which is what I endeavor to do, but yes, it is a painful, emotional experience at times.

Psalm 147:5 is one of my favorite verses: "Great is our Lord, and of great power: his understanding is infinite."

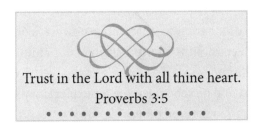

Trust in the Lord with all thine heart.
Proverbs 3:5

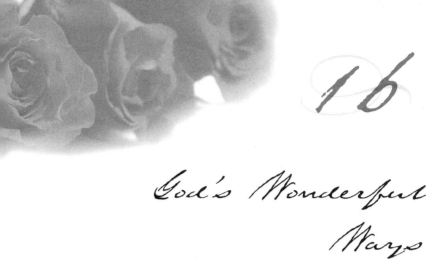

16

God's Wonderful Ways

—*anonymous*

WE WERE ONLY married for six months when I discovered I was expecting a baby. My husband and I were attempting to adjust to marriage as well as the financial obligations which come along with marriage. Consequently, I struggled with the idea of a child coming so quickly.

When I went to the doctor for the initial visit, I was probably seven weeks along. The nurse asked me many questions. She asked if I had any pain or cramping. I had experienced a fair amount, but I assured her I had avoided any medication. Someone (the nurse or the doctor) insisted I go for an ultrasound that same day.

The doctor came in following the ultrasound and informed me that my baby was not in the uterus. He told me I would need emergency surgery that day. I stopped at my husband's work place and informed him of the situation.

I had surgery that afternoon. The doctor used a laser and was able to save my tube. It was also determined during that surgery that I have endometriosis. Much of the endometriosis was removed, but the probability of having children remained unknown.

I remember feeling tired and sore for about two weeks after the surgery. Emotionally, I had my ups and downs. I felt guilty because I was not very excited about having a baby. I felt scared that I would never be able to have any more children. It was the first real traumatic experience for our new marriage. Overall, it was a little rough.

Two months later, I discovered I was pregnant again! I raced to the doctor for an ultrasound. Thankfully, everything was in its right place this time. The following May, I gave birth to a healthy baby boy. A little over two years later, another boy was added to our family. Twenty months went by and boy number three arrived. I must admit my nervousness about another ectopic pregnancy had gone. I had three normal pregnancies, so I must be "okay."

Time went by and boy number three had his first birthday, and I had my first cycle. About two or three weeks later, on a Saturday, I had terrible abdominal pain. It was so bad I had to lie down. I told my husband I might need to go to the ER. We placed a call to the doctor. As I lay there and waited for his return call, I decided I need to have to bowel movement. I painfully hobbled to the bathroom. I felt so much relief afterwards. I still felt tender, sore and bloated, but didn't have as much pain. When the doctor called back, he told me to go to the ER if the pain resumed. If not, I was to see him in his office on Monday.

I was able to make it until Monday. I noticed additional bloating along with continued tenderness. The doctor's office routinely performed a pregnancy test. I was shocked when it came back positive! I had just had my cycle! I knew then that something was definitely not right. We went to our local hospital for an ultrasound.

When we were still in the waiting room, following the scan, my doctor called the nurse at the desk. She called me to the phone. The doctor told me I had another ectopic pregnancy. I stayed at the hospital, where they prepared me for another surgery.

Surprisingly, it was in my other tube! The doctor had to remove most of that tube. I had been bleeding a little internally, which explained the bloating. Now I was left with only one tube which had already been operated on. Would we be able to have any more children?

My husband and I wanted another child, but we decided a little space might be good. Our home was very active. My husband worked long hours. It was dangerous for me to get pregnant. Could I even get pregnant again? I tried to keep track of my ovulation for several months. With this one month, two weeks went past my expected day of ovulation. I thought I must have missed it.

Well, God has wonderful ways beyond our human minds. He made my body ovulate two weeks late so I could conceive again. Boy number four blessed our home nine months later. I continue to marvel at God's power. First, I really shouldn't have been able to conceive because of the damaged tube and the endometriosis. Secondly, I was watching my cycle. I knew that this child was a special gift from God.

Boy number four was born a perfect baby. We enjoyed the first month of his life. At about six weeks, we noticed a rash appear. His condition declined. At five months, he was diagnosed with a rare disease which is treated with chemotherapy somewhat like cancer. I have gone back to the special miracle of his conception many times. I have found comfort in the assurance that God had a plan for his life.

Our family struggled with living with a child who had a

chronic life-threatening disease. He was immune suppressed much of the time, so we kept him away from groups of people. We felt our family was pulled apart, as some would go to church or a family gathering, while leaving one parent and boy number four at home. It was difficult.

I discovered baby number five was on the way when baby number four was about to turn two. Even though I was amazed that I could conceive with only one previously operated on tube, I wondered how I would deal with occasional hospital stays and weekly chemo treatments for boy number four, not to mention the other three young boys who needed me.

Yes, baby number five was a boy, too! I am so thankful to God that He has blessed us with five beautiful children.

We haven't had any additional children, so the ectopic story ends here. We were disappointed when boy number five was diagnosed with cerebral palsy. Then, on March 8, 2006, God took our angel, boy number four, home to Heaven. God will lead us into tomorrow and take care of our needs then as well.

There are days of silent sorrow
in the seasons of our life,
There are wild, despairing moments,
and the never-ending strife.
There are times of stony anguish
when the tears refuse to fall,
But the waiting time, my friends,
is the hardest time of all.

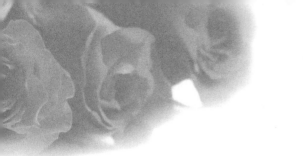

17

Little Miracle

—*Brian & Marnita Wennerstrom, Belmont, OH*

IT WAS JULY of 2005, and we had just celebrated our only child's first birthday. My menstrual cycle had returned postpartum, but it was irregular at best. We thought nothing of it when I began to bleed. I spotted through about five days. On Friday evening we decided to go to the The Living Word, a Christian outdoor drama. I had not been having a very good day and the evening wasn't shaping up so well either. Our son was fussy, bees stung me twice, and then the cramping started. I commented to my husband that maybe it was a tubal pregnancy, but I quickly dismissed the thought, thinking the pain was not severe enough. I lay curled up in a fetal position for the duration of the trip home. I still thought it was normal. By the time we arrived home, the cramping had let up a little, and with some Tylenol I was able to rest.

When Monday afternoon arrived, things had not gotten much better, and my husband convinced me to take a pregnancy test. I was 90% sure I wasn't pregnant. I was having my period—how could I be? Well, the test showed positive, but the line on the test indicating pregnancy was faint. We called my OB/GYN, wondering what we should do. She advised us to either go to a nearby emergency room or come directly to her office, nearly two hours away. We decided to make the longer trip to someone we trusted. They told us, "Pack some clothes—we may need to do surgery tonight." My mind was reeling and my heart was in denial. I wanted to hope for the best. I had just found out I was pregnant! This was supposed to be a time for happiness and rejoicing. I wanted this baby. I wanted to linger in the joy of the beginning; not think about the fact that it was ending...so very soon.

As I hurriedly threw things into the suitcase, words from a song were running through my head: "God is in control/ We believe that His children will not be forsaken/God is in control/We will choose to remember and never be shaken/ There is no power above or beside Him we know/God is in control."

When we arrived at the doctor's, an ultrasound showed there was nothing in my uterus, but there was fluid behind it. The fluid was blood that had begun leaking into my abdominal cavity. The doctor didn't need any more confirmation. She told us to head for the hospital, where she would do surgery immediately. I cried as I gave my mom instructions for the care of our one-year-old. This would be the first time I was separated from our son for overnight. He was still breast-feeding and especially dependent on me for sleeping.

Later that night I was being prepped for surgery. The emotionally packed evening had taken its toll on me and I was tired. My husband's presence in the pre-surgery room was very comforting. As they wheeled me to the operating room, I prayed for strength to combat the anxiety that wanted to overwhelm me. I shivered with the reality of what they were about to do and the freezing temperatures of the operating room. In the surgery the doctor found that my tube had not burst, and thus she was able to save it. Inside the tube she found the placenta but nothing remaining of the baby. I must have been five or six weeks along. We praise the Lord for causing us to take the pregnancy test when we did. Hours or days later could have produced a very different outcome.

My grief became very real in the weeks that followed. I felt I had lost someone very special. Most people around me acknowledged our loss in the best way they knew how. As Christians, we say that life begins at conception, but the indifference of some to our loss made us wonder if they *really* believed it. I struggled to not take it personally. My experience has led me to realize that when a mother loses a baby, at any stage in the pregnancy, she needs comfort and encouragement. I know I did. I

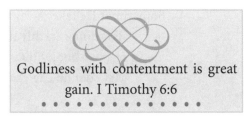

Godliness with contentment is great gain. I Timothy 6:6

cherished every word, every phone call, every lovingly written card I received.

It seemed that so many friends, including my own sister, were pregnant and due around the same time I would have been. It was hard for me to leave it all in God's hands. I knew there was a possibility that scar tissue could make conception difficult. I also realized that my chances for a tubal pregnancy had increased. A practical way we deal with that worry is to take a pregnancy test every time I bleed (even though I'm sure it's just my period). Pregnancy tests have become a staple at our house. In the midst of my worries, God began forming another "little miracle." Almost a year later, I gave birth to a beautiful, healthy boy, who is now almost eight months old. God is good!

We framed a card from a friend with a lovely drawing of Jesus holding a baby in a rocking chair. It has a special place in our nursery as a beautiful reminder that all innocent life God creates (including our little one), He takes Home to be with Him at the moment of death. That is comforting indeed.

Soaring

Sometimes God takes away our props
That we might lean on Him,
Allows temptations, so we'll grow
And triumph over sin.

Sometimes He takes away our strength
For doing earthly things
To rest our bodies that our souls
May soar on eagle's wings.

Let's not resent it when He says,
"Come ye apart—be still,"
Or chafe at disappointments
That are His sovereign will.

Oh, let's not doubt or question "why?"
With unexplained delays,
And keep on soaring 'neath His wings
With gratitude and praise!

—*Author Unknown*

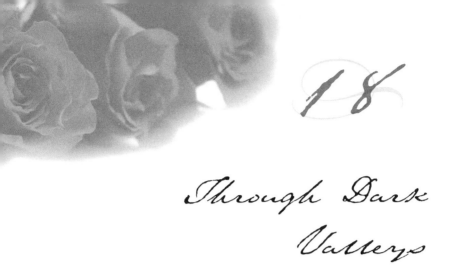

Through Dark Valleys

—Wilbur & Anita Wampler, Chambersburg, PA

WILBUR AND I have been married for thirteen years. I had two miscarriages first, which were very hard to accept, especially when my two brothers were married after us and were having children with no problems. These pregnancies were lost by the time we knew I was even pregnant, so we really didn't have dashed hopes, other than knowing that we had lost what we really wanted—children.

At this point I was having my hopes high, just to be dashed at the start of each period. After being married three years my third pregnancy ended up to be my first tubal.

We were working with a doctor who was trying to help us find our problem as to why it was so hard for me to conceive. He had me on Clomid to help me get pregnant and then progesterone for the second half of my cycle. I was already taking Clomid the next month when I started having pain on my left side and started to bleed. The doctor said it was just an irregular period and didn't worry about it.

To say the least, I was worried because of my history and couldn't get the discomfort out of my mind. We as a couple prayed and tried to accept that the doctor knew what was right.

After a couple days we went in to the doctor's office because of the pain, and they sent me to the hospital to take a sonogram, which didn't show anything out of the ordinary. We went back to the doctor's office, and on the way there we prayed for God's mercy. I still knew there was something wrong with me and prayed that God would help them find the problem. Wilbur was a comfort by just being there and helping to ease my worries and praying for me.

The doctor decided to do an internal exam, and when I nearly hit the ceiling fan when he tried, he knew that I was not a fake. He left the room and went to talk to his partner and when he came back he said he wanted to do exploratory surgery. He set the surgery up for the next day and told us what to expect and what to do.

We had our families praying for us, and it was such a comfort to know that God cared and that we had many people interceding to God on our behalf.

The next day I wasn't to eat or drink for a while before the surgery, and when we got there he had another emergency surgery, so I had to wait longer. They, in the meantime, were getting me ready for the operation, and Wilbur was by my side, encouraging me.

When I finally got into surgery, they found a pregnancy in the tube which they took out, without taking the tube. The whole surgery turned out well, but I remember the uncertainty of the procedure and the feelings afterward about taking a pregnancy that was growing and getting rid of it. I really struggled with that part of an ectopic pregnancy. I thought to myself that they can do so many things; why can't they remove an ectopic pregnancy and implant it in the womb?

I was originally supposed to go home that same day, but

when things got late and my one incision was seeping, I had to stay overnight. I just wanted to go home and leave the struggles behind. Wilbur slept on a chair in the room with me, and early the next morning I was discharged.

When we got home we went through a lot of up and down emotions. It seemed like our hopes of having children were slowly disintegrating.

One of the things we struggled with was people saying things like, "You're still young yet; just give yourself a little more time" or "Just relax and you will get pregnant." We found that if you want to be a follower of Jesus, you need to have a lot of forgiveness for people, even friends. We realized that they were only trying to comfort us in our state of disappointment, but some of the statements were more harmful than helpful.

We want to say that there were a lot of people who really knew how to show love. We still hold their love and concern in our hearts and are challenged by their deeds of kindness. We hope that our lives can touch some other person in their hour of need. One song that touched our lives through our struggles was, "Does Jesus Care?"

My second ectopic pregnancy (which was after having another miscarriage) was much the same. In fact, so much the same that when we arrived at the hospital, we walked in and told the lady at the front desk that we were sure that I was having a tubal pregnancy. They asked me when I had my last period. When I told them it was two weeks before and that I do not miss my period when I am pregnant, they just dismissed the idea, thinking I didn't know what I was talking about.

After several people asked me the same questions and got the same answer from me (all of them looking at me in a funny way), they decided to take a sonogram to see if they could find the problem. They knew my symptoms pointed towards my assumption being right, but the period date didn't make sense.

When the sonogram was read by the doctor, they told me I was going straight to the operating table because I was bleeding internally. When they all left the room for a little while, we had a short prayer that the Lord would protect me again and that He would guide the doctor's hands. I told Wilbur that I didn't want to go through this again, but I was ready for relief. Before we parted, Wilbur gave me encouragement and a hug and a kiss. In fifteen minutes I was wheeled into the operating room, and the last thing I remember was everyone rushing around.

Wilbur left and went to get something to eat while I was having the operation. He called my parents to send the news around our church calling chain to ask for prayer. He also called one of our close friends and told him I was going through another ectopic pregnancy. He unloaded his feelings to him and asked for their prayers.

When I became conscious, Wilbur soon came in to see me. The first thing that came to my mind was, *Thank you, Jesus, that we can still be together.* They told us that everything went well, even though I had lost a lot of blood. They had to take the tube, but there was no need to give me blood. We had something to praise God for, but as the next weeks unfolded, like normal, I was the first to hit low times.

Wilbur always seemed to be able to encourage me when I was struggling. Then as I felt like I was getting to the point of accepting another disappointment, then Wilbur would hit his low point. I think he felt it was his responsibility to help me through, then he allowed his real feelings to surface. I thank God that He gave me a husband that could take the pressures, and that we weren't both down at the same time. When he hit his low time I tried to encourage him, but sometimes it was almost like it tried to drag me down with him. We always knew that God had a reason for everything in our lives, and that He is always right and just, no matter whether we understand or not. This is one thing that Wilbur reminded me of very often, and I am glad to have a husband who has such convictions and beliefs.

This loss was a real faith trial for us. Right after we came home from the hospital, we went to see my parents. My mother was the only one at home, and Wilbur, feeling under stress, broke down and told my mother he felt like God was teasing us like an adult that would tease a child with candy, and then never give it to them. We went home with our frustrations, but knew my mother would go straight to her room, get on her knees, and pray for us in our struggles. Just that fact soon broke Wilbur's anger, and he called her back soon and told her he was sorry for talking about God in that way. We understand now that God was just bringing us through some trials to strengthen our faith in Him and our belief that He is always just.

I felt weak from loss of blood, and had lots of pain after the operation. Our church sisters sent us meals every other day for several weeks. I had to have someone help me move around for several days and I slept on the recliner several nights. I was not supposed to do any heavy lifting for a while, and I didn't feel like eating for a couple days.

Two years later,

My help cometh from the Lord, which made heaven and earth.
Psalm 121:2

we had a stillborn at five months. This was one of the hardest yet easiest losses. Hardest because we thought we were past the problem stage and in the clear, but easiest because we knew that it was in God's plan. He wanted us to pass the tests He was sending.

After being married over ten years, we started into adoption, which took until we were married twelve years and one month to get finalized. We now have two sons, ages three and five, who are such a blessing and challenge in our lives. After having them in our home for ten months, I started having pain on the way home from our anniversary trip to the cabin. We had promised the boys (we had taken them along because they were not used to being left behind and we were still trying to fully bond with them) some ice cream.

By the time Wilbur came out of the restaurant, I was in severe pain. There were some things different, like no bleeding, and I didn't know what to think. The pain came and went in its severity, so it was a couple of days later that I finally went to my doctor. He sent me to the hospital to get blood drawn for a pregnancy test and to check for infection.

When we got back to his office, he had gotten the test for the infection, which was positive. He suspected I had another ectopic pregnancy and sent me straight back to the hospital. When I got back they took me in and started to get all my information to take me as an outpatient. The nurse said something about me being pregnant, to which I answered, "I don't know," for I had not yet known the test results.

Some time later another man came and told us that I did have another ectopic pregnancy. I would be having surgery as soon as they had a room ready for me. I was having more pain all the while and was struggling with the fact that I was having still another pregnancy, and would be spending more money for seemingly nothing profitable. We were left to sit for at least two hours while they did this and that, getting things ready for surgery.

Finally a very kind nurse came and started to push me down the hall. I was relieved to be getting that close to relief from the sharp pain I was enduring, when another nurse came and wondered if I'm Anita. We told her, "Yes."

"Well, I have bad news. The doctor was called to deliver a baby and it will be a little while until he can come." I felt like I had been smacked square in the face. Someone was about to have the joy of their life fulfilled, while I had to wait in pain for disappointment to be accomplished in my life.

I felt like crying my heart out. *Why, God, did you do this to me?* It's hard enough without extra tests planted in the path I was to walk. I spilled my feelings to Wilbur, and he tried to encourage me in the love of God. He told me that things are not always fair, but God does not ask us to walk where He can not carry us through. We had another prayer to help calm our discomforts.

About twenty minutes later, they came to get me for the second time. Wilbur came with me as far as he could, then we said our good-byes and exchanged our encouragements. The doctor told us what would happen, which by now we were already familiar with. He told us how he would take the other tube because of the many ectopic pregnancies I had. He told Wilbur where he could spend the next hour and a half while he waited for me.

The next thing he asked, we were not familiar with from a doctor. "I like to pray with all my patients before we go into the operating room. Is that okay?" We readily agreed and everyone bowed their heads while he had a silent moment of prayer. Then I was taken to the operating room once again. As they started to give me anesthesia, the song "Lo, I Come" was going through my mind.

Lo, I Come

Lo, I come to do Thy will, O God, I come;
By Thy Spirit let me dwell, O God, I come.

Keep me sober and sincere, O God, I come;
Let not Satan interfere, O God, I come.

Loving Father, take my hand, O God, I come;
Lead me to that Heavenly land, O God, I come.

Chorus:
Walk beside me and guide me;
Help me daily to be holy;
Oh, I need Thee, yes, I plead Thee,
Let me live to Thy praise,
Let me walk in Thy ways.

When the operation was over the doctor came and told me he had saved the tube after all because of how perfect it looked. I had mixed feelings in my grogginess about having the tube saved. *Thank you, God* that I had not lost all my femininity, but *Oh, no! I might have to go through this again!*

The doctor next showed Wilbur some pictures and said that my body had actually expelled the pregnancy from the tube on its own. I was not allowed to go home that evening, so Wilbur drove home after midnight, close to a two-hour drive, and came back the next day to take me home.

It took several days to recuperate till I could handle my sons at home. It was hard for me to see how hard they took it, not being with us. We have learned a lot and have grown through the experiences we went through. We feel that without these tests in life we would not be the people we are today and our faith would be weak. We thank and praise God for all He has brought us through by His power. A few of the songs that meant a lot to us through our tough times are these:

Life is easy when you're up on the mountain
And you've got peace of mind, like you've never known,
Then things change and you're down in the valley,
Don't lose faith for you're never alone.

For the God of the mountain is still God in the valley,
When things go wrong He'll make them right,
And the God of the good times is still God in the bad times.
The God of the day is still God in the night.

We talk of faith when we're up on the mountain,
But talk comes so easy when life's at its best,
But it's down in the valley of trials and temptations
That's when faith is really put to the test.

My God I Thank Thee

My God, I thank Thee who hast made
	the earth so bright
So full of splendor and of joy
	beauty and light
So many glorious things are here
	noble and right.

I thank Thee, too, that Thou hast made
    joy to abound
So many gentle thoughts and deeds
    circling us round
That in the darkest spot of earth
    some love is found.

I thank Thee more that all our joy
    is touched with pain
That shadows fall on brightest hours
    that thorns remain
So that earth's bliss may be our guide
    and not our chain.

I thank Thee, Lord, that Thou hast kept
    the best in store
We have enough yet not too much
    to long for more
A yearning for a deeper peace
    not known before.

The last verse of this song is the reason we can sing the third verse with confidence through our times of testing. Praise the Lord for His everlasting love and kindness toward man.

Now no chastening for the present seemeth to be joyous, but grievous: nevertheless afterward it yieldeth the peaceable fruit of righteouness unto them which are exercised thereby. Hebrews 12:11

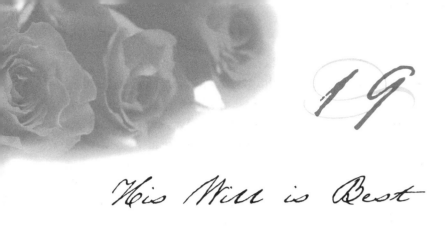

19

His Will is Best

—*anonymous*

MY HEART BEAT fast as I laid the pregnancy test on a flat surface to await the results. My period was late, and I was hoping against hope that I might finally be pregnant again.

My husband and I had been married for two years, and so far God had not blessed us with children. An earlier pregnancy had ended in miscarriage, to our great disappointment and grief. After all these months it seemed almost too good to be true that I could really be pregnant again.

And sure enough, after three minutes the test was negative. Disgusted, I threw the test into a drawer and went my way. Later, I again picked up the test and being in a brighter room this time, I noticed a very faint positive mark. However, knowing that you aren't supposed to read results after half an hour, and also thinking such a faint line could not be positive, we decided that, once again, I wasn't pregnant.

However, I still didn't get my period.

A couple days later was the wedding of my husband's brother. His wife-to-be lived in another state, and we were planning a trip to attend. That night we had to get up at 1:00 a.m. to be ready in time for our van. My period still had not started, and since I am a very regular, 28-day person, this was rather unusual. I had one test left and decided to use it. Then, to my disbelieving eyes, there it was—a positive sign!

Immediately I called my husband, who came over and looked at the test. But to him, the possibility that I could actually be pregnant was so remote that at first he was sure the test was wrong! Looking back, it amuses me, but really, I had some of the same feelings. After trying so hard for so long, it just didn't seem possible that it had finally happened again. We were overjoyed, and truly felt God was answering our prayers. And for me, the wedding day was even more enjoyable with the thought of a precious baby on the way.

However, after we came back home again and into daily routine, the worries came. I was desperately afraid this baby would also be taken from us through miscarriage. (Later, we found ourselves thinking, "If only it had been *just* a miscarriage.")

I tried to take care, but it was spring and a very busy time, with field, garden and yard work. With only my husband and me to keep after things, I found it almost impossible to take care as I wished.

Daily I fought this giant of worry. My husband felt that this time everything would work out, and encouraged me not to borrow trouble or worry before there is a reason, but to trust more. Wise words of advice, but it seemed I was almost unable to do so. When we knelt to pray, the only words that came were, "Please, God, let us keep this baby if it is Your will."

And God, in His all-knowing wisdom and wonderful love, for reasons that we cannot yet understand, chose to take this baby from us also.

One morning when I awoke, to my utmost dismay, I discovered that I was spotting. I think we both knew right away that there was no hope.

An immediate call was made to our midwife, who advised us to go for an ultrasound, so that we don't need to go through the suspense of waiting to see whether or not a miscarriage would occur. At this point, we just figured that's what is happening, although I had also thought of a tubal pregnancy. Mainly because my cousin had one just a couple of months earlier, and her story was still fresh in my mind. But also because, in looking over the symptoms of miscarriages and tubal pregnancies, I noticed "brown spotting" listed as a sign of a tubal pregnancy. This was what I had.

I spent the majority of that day in the easy chair. We decided not to go for an ultrasound, figuring that if it is a miscarriage, it would likely soon be over, like it had been the first time I miscarried.

By the next morning my condition had not changed. I was still spotting, but not more than I had been the day before. I was suddenly very ready to find out what was going on. I felt I could not bear sitting around, waiting to see what will happen.

We managed to get an appointment for that forenoon yet, and soon I found myself lying on a table, awaiting the ultrasound. How I hoped to see a flickering heartbeat, and be told that everything looks fine, and that I only have "normal spotting." But, of course, that was not to be.

The technician probed around for a long time, first on one side, then on the other. Finally I asked her if she can see anything.

"Well, I can see nothing in the uterus," she answered, "and as far as you are along, I should be able to see something."

"Is there a possibility that it's in the tube?" I wondered shakily. She put her hand on my shoulder and gently told me there was. She then went to speak with my doctor, and I was left sitting in a cold, dim room, fearful of what was going on. How I wished for the supportive presence of my husband, who, because of farm work, had not accompanied me.

After what seemed like a long time, the lady returned, and it was decided that I would come again on Monday. This was Friday, so that left a long, long weekend to live through.

I had many phantom pains those two days, and once I called the doctor and told her I'm not sure if I dare wait any longer to do something. She asked me how bad the pain is, on a scale of one to ten. "Well," I said, "if I wasn't afraid I have a tubal pregnancy, I probably would think nothing of it." Naturally, her advice was, "Don't worry."

Finally Monday arrived, and that has probably been the first time I've been glad to go to the doctor! It turned out to be a very long, very stressful day. Once there, a more experienced lady did the ultrasound, and again, there was nothing in the uterus. But she spotted a small dark blob on my right tube. The doctor confirmed my suspicions that it was, indeed, a tubal pregnancy.

Then, following a few bewildering hours of hospitals, blood tests, doctors, etc., I was given the option of doing surgery or trying medication. Again, I wished fervently for my husband. Since we hadn't realized what all would be involved, he again had chosen not to come with me.

I chose to try the medication, as it was so much cheaper and easier than surgery, and would also save my tube if it worked properly. I was given two shots of Methotrexate, which is really a form of chemotherapy. In plain words, the purpose of this was to dissolve our baby. Oh, what a feeling—the baby we so much wanted! And yet there was just nothing we could do about it.

How glad I was to come home that day, to my own familiar house and dear husband. And what a relief to let go of all the emotions I had been holding in check all day.

We were told that the medication might not work, and my tube could still rupture at any time. If I had shoulder pain,

pain in my side, nausea, dizziness or a fainting feeling, I should head to the nearest emergency room. This was complicated by the fact that the shots gave me stomach pain, and it was difficult to know whether or not it was serious. The shots also made me bleed heavily. (I actually bled for a whole month before finally stopping.)

I had no work limitations, but I didn't feel well, and was glad for help with the heavier work. My husband had to shoulder all the barn chores, which added more stress to his already busy days.

Two days after the shots, my shoulder started hurting. Whether it truly was pain, or the result of an overactive imagination, I cannot say. However, I panicked, and called the doctor. They asked me to come in for an ultrasound, which showed the blob had shrunken already—a good sign. I relaxed and that night I slept without the fear that I would awaken in terrible pain with a ruptured tube.

The shots called for a lot of follow-up blood work, so four days later, I had to have my HCG levels checked. They had dropped from 2,500 to about 1,500. We relaxed further. After all, we had been told that in 80-90% of cases Methotrexate works.

A week after the shots, I again went to have my levels checked. That afternoon the nurse called with the results, and they were not good. My levels were back up to 2,600.

She told me I need to come to their pharmacy and get more medication, then go to their hospital's emergency room (40 miles away) for a repeat shot. It was Sunday afternoon, we had company, and it was almost chore

Why should I worry;
God knows the way;
He knows each tomorrow,
As well as today.

time. We didn't know *what* to do.

I begged the nurse to find a pharmacy closer to us that would carry it. I thought maybe then our midwife could give me the shots, and I wouldn't have to go to the hospital. The nurse went beyond her call of duty and so kindly called all the pharmacies closer to us, all to no avail, however. They were all either closed or did not carry it. I then asked if I would just get it at their pharmacy then let the midwife give the shots to avoid an emergency room bill. The nurse thought that could work if the doctor and the midwife talked with each other.

We were told this is the last chance before surgery, because if two shots don't work, three won't either. Many anxious hours were in store for us as we waited to find out if it is working this time. The fear of my tube rupturing was always with us, and there were many nights I was almost afraid to go to sleep.

My next blood work showed my levels had dropped to around 2,400. We had hoped for a bigger drop, but were assured that this is fine.

By now I was feeling well physically, and back to doing my own work. By far the worst part was the stress and uncertainty of wondering what's going to happen.

During this time I was almost paranoid about going away. I remember once my mother had gone with me when I went for some blood work, and we also did some shopping. I was sure I would suddenly drop to the floor with a ruptured tube. I guess such fears were irrational, but at the time they were very real.

I kept going for blood work, and my levels dropped to 1,400, then to 500. Now, surely, we thought, everything should be all right. The doctors had impressed on our minds how important it is to have a 30% drop in the first week after the shots, but what they did not talk much about was the fact that my tube could still rupture till my levels were at 0.

But—it did appear to be working. My last blood work had

been on a Saturday, and that Sunday we finally dared to go to church again. My husband's parents had the reception for their newly married son, so we were there that afternoon. I felt well, almost back to normal.

That night I slept well and awoke feeling fine. But soon after breakfast I became aware that not all is well. I had an ill feeling, and pressure in my abdomen. This quickly became worse. It felt like I had a bladder infection or a very full bladder, when in fact I didn't.

Soon I started feeling light-headed and nauseated. I remember so clearly going out and sitting on the porch, sure that I would either faint or throw up any minute. I did neither, but my head kept buzzing. For awhile I had a burning sensation on my right side, but this soon disappeared.

We were both scared and unsure of what we should do. We didn't know if we should rush to the emergency room or if it wasn't even serious. My husband called the doctor, and like usual, had to leave a message. Other times our call was returned immediately, but this time, of all times, they didn't. In desperation, my husband paged the doctor, which in turn produced a call from a rather irritated nurse, who wondered how in the world we knew the pager number. (Another nurse had given it earlier.)

At least we got the attention we needed so much, and we were told to come in for an ultrasound. The memory of my husband, helping his bent-over wife get dressed to go to the doctor, makes me smile now, but at the time it wasn't funny.

Lying on the table at the doctor's office, I suddenly felt much better, and already felt foolish, coming in again, as I thought, about nothing.

The technician said she sees extra fluid, but when we asked what that means, she just said she needs to talk with the doctor. They took me in to see her, and her first words were, "No, you don't look very well, do you?" She examined me, and with the evidence of the ultrasound she informed us that I need surgery that day yet.

It was around 1:00, and she said she would finish her office hours and do the surgery around 6:00. When we asked what went wrong that I still needed surgery, she had no answer for us. She only told us that it goes like this sometimes, and that it was a good pregnancy in the wrong place.

We then went to the hospital. There we had a couple hours' wait yet. I was so thankful for my husband's calm presence, as I felt terrified of having surgery. I dreaded being put to sleep and imagined how it would be to get drowsier and drowsier, and realizing that I was being "put out." A useless worry, as it wasn't like that at all.

When the nurses came to put an IV line in my hand, they had quite a struggle. I normally have small veins in my hands, and since I was cold and shivering (partly from nerves) my veins were even smaller. They stuck me a couple of times with no success. This was very painful, and left black and blue marks. Finally they went to the crook of my arm, where they managed to get it in.

I was wheeled off to the operating room and given a tranquilizer, which made my brain spin. I also remember someone reaching over my head and injecting something into my IV line.

The next thing I knew, I was back in my room, with my husband sitting beside me. It was around 10:00 p.m. The doctor had told him that my abdomen had been full of blood, hence the pressure. The tube had been bleeding out of the end. To this day I don't know whether it would eventually have ruptured if they hadn't removed it, or if they were afraid the bleeding wouldn't stop.

We wanted to go home that night yet, if possible. But first I had to take a walk down the hall. I felt so wobbly and light-headed, but desperately wanted to go home. How endless that hall looked! I, for some reason, thought I must walk the full length of it.

After a couple yards, when the nurse asked if I want to go back now, I was like "you mean this was far enough?!" After eating something and not getting nauseated, I was discharged.

Our faithful driver and friend who had brought us to the hospital had waited for us all those hours, even though she was more than half sick with a bad cold, and did not like to drive in the dark. Again, I feel this was God helping us through a person. How can you ever adequately thank someone for something you appreciated so much??

The day after surgery I was groggy and disoriented. All I wanted to do was sleep and sleep.

I was supposed to take it easy for two weeks, and kind relatives came to help out the first week. By the next week I was back to doing my own work. I paid for it by being exhausted, but by the end of that week I felt better than I had since before the whole thing began.

I had to go for one checkup, and to get my stitches out. Then, suddenly, the whole ordeal ended.

After I no longer spent my energies being concerned about myself, the emotional pain set in. This was also hard on my husband; much harder than our previous loss had been.

Added to the loss of our baby was the loss of most of my fertility. In addition to having my tube removed, the surgery revealed that I have endometriosis, a common fertility problem. It would appear that our chances of having another child are very slim.

As I am writing this, it is five days before our baby's due date would have been. How our hearts ached this month. Sometimes it has almost seemed overwhelming. But what a comfort to think of our two beautiful babies in Heaven! Truly they are so much better off there than they would be had they come to this earth.

We have many days when we must struggle with anger and bitterness. Why us? But always, there is the thought that this did not just *happen;* it was the will of God. And while we don't understand now, maybe sometime we will. Then likely we will thank God from the bottom of our hearts for allowing it to be so.

And too, we often think that it could be so much worse. There are so many sick and grieving people, and those who live in poverty, in war-torn countries, and those in the sin-filled world. Thinking along these lines, it is not hard to count our blessings. Indeed, why us? Why are we so blessed?

Of course, we hope that someday a miracle will occur and we will yet be blessed with a precious baby, either by birth or adoption.

But God's plans are not always ours, and we don't know what the future holds. We can only ask for grace and strength to bear what comes, for God does help carry the burdens He gives. We want to accept God's will and be content.

> In whatsoever our lot may be,
> Calmly in this thought we'll rest,
> Could we see as Thou dost see,
> We would choose it as the best.

And may we all keep on striving so that hopefully some day, by the grace of God, we will be able to meet our babies in Heaven.

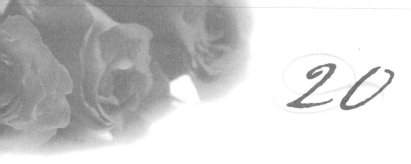

20

The Unknown Future

—*Ruth Overholt, Minerva, OH*

THE LORD TAKES us through fiery trials and many different things. We want to ask, "why?", but knowing the Lord is in control is a real consolation.

My sister and I have both had tubal pregnancies. The doctor said with us both having one does not mean it is hereditary. All our mother's pregnancies were normal. My sister and I are the only girls in a family of eight.

My sister was about two months along when she had pretty serious bleeding and severe pain so that she couldn't walk. When she got to the hospital, they discovered a tubal pregnancy that had already burst. She had to have the tube removed on that side. She was in the hospital about five days and had to have a blood transfusion. Some people told her she would only be able to have one gender if she got pregnant again. But she had a boy and two girls afterwards.

My experience took place in October of 1997. I started spotting and thought it was only my period. But I just kept on bleeding, and with my sister's experience, I was on the alert! I talked to my OB-GYN doctor's nurse. She asked me to do a pregnancy test. This was on October 9, and it showed positive. She told me to come in for a checkup. The next day I had to go in for a transvaginal ultrasound, but they couldn't find anything.

Blood work was done on the 10th, 12th and 14th. The HCG count had been up, but went down again. The lab technician told me that the baby could hardly be living anymore. On the 15th I called some of my sisters-in-law and told them I think it is all over. I felt I was miscarrying the baby, due to my heavy bleeding and clotting.

Around 4:00 that same day, the doctor called and said the last blood count went up again. He wanted me at the hospital by 6:00 p.m. The doctor was questioning a tubal, but the only symptoms were bleeding. He said he would do an exploratory laparoscopy to see what's going on.

My body was shaking from the shock and fear of the unknown. My prayers went out to God for reassurance and guidance. I had to make phone calls to my husband at work and also to a sister-in-law to take care of our three girls.

By the time we got to the hospital at 6:30 p.m., I was calmer and placed my trust and my body into the hands of God and the doctors. Around 9:45 I was given anesthesia, and woke up around 1:00 a.m. The doctor had told us that if it's in the tube, there isn't anything they can do to save the baby. It was a tubal and the doctor slit the tube and it fell out. They also did a D&C right away. I had a total of three small incisions.

The doctor gave me pictures of the bulging tube. We were so thankful it was taken care of before it burst. The doctor left the tube in and told me if I would have another tubal in the same tube, they would remove all the organs on that side. They advised me not to get pregnant for a year, and once I did, I would have to come for an ultrasound to make sure everything is okay.

I got pregnant in the fall of 1998. I had an ultrasound done, but I had to have the second one done a couple days later before it showed in the uterus. I gave birth to our first son on May 26, 1999.

In June of 2003, I experienced a miscarriage. I feared it might be another tubal. They did an ultrasound, but couldn't find anything. Once my HCG blood count started coming down, it kept dropping to where the doctor thought it should be okay without doing a D&C.

After my tubal pregnancy it took me about a week to get over the tenderness from surgery. It was when I was healing well physically that I was hit most with the loss of a precious child. The grief seemed greater with my miscarriage. We were saddened with the loss in the tubal, but at the same time, very aware of the fact that my life could also have been taken. Going through these experiences makes us so much more thankful for the four healthy children God gave us, and with the accident our two oldest were in, that the Lord let us have them with us for some time longer. (At the time of this writing, it is a week since our two oldest daughters were in a bad car accident. They were both hurt badly and had blood on the brain.) We count it a blessing and miracle upon miracles that we still have them with us.

Our biggest consolation throughout everything we experienced is that the Lord is the one who created us and cares for us. He knows what He wants for us and He will carry it out.

We have so much to be thankful for and we want the Lord to continue to lead us through the unknown future.

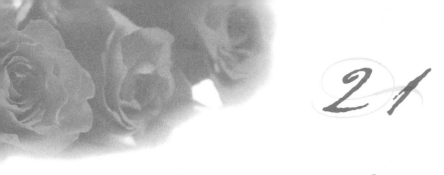

21

A Birthday Trial

—*Allen & Eleanor Zimmerman, Penn Yan, NY*

WE LIVED ON a dairy farm and had a family of two healthy children, a happy two-year-old Anthony and nine-month-old Carolyn. I was 32 years old and blessed with good health. I learned a lot through this experience, as God is Almighty and in everything there is a purpose.

I had a normal period on December 27, 1998, but the next one I skipped. Up until February 6th I felt fine, but on that day I felt pressure on my lower right side. Later it sort of dulled.

On Sunday we went to church, then to a friend's house for dinner. After dinner the pain returned, but not bad enough to mention it to anyone. My husband brought in a tiny miniature collie puppy with a big red ribbon, a birthday surprise for me. She was too young to take home yet, which was good, as I'd have to spend time in the hopsital that night yet. But it did give me something to look forward to.

Around midnight the pain became worse, so we decided to go to the hospital. We suspected it might be appendicitis. The roads were bad and snow was falling, with twelve to fifteen inches on the ground already. We called the ambulance and asked for a ride to the hospital, with no sirens or much fuss, as we felt it's not an emergency.

My husband's sister wasn't in bed yet, as her special

friend had just left for home. She came and stayed with the children.

To our surprise about a dozen or so volunteers came. Many of them asked us the same questions and wrote them on their paper. It seemed as if they were taking training lessons. We almost wished we wouldn't have called.

It was early Monday morning, on February 8th, my birthday, that we arrived at the hospital. Pain had settled in my lower right side. An ultrasound showed fluid in my tube and a suspicious mass, which was proof of an ectopic, instead of appendicitis, as we had thought. I was given a painkiller which helped a lot.

Since Penn Yan couldn't handle this type of surgery, they tried to send me to Geneva. But the doctors there couldn't agree or get along very well, so they tried the hospital in Canandaigua. Dr. Cant agreed to accept another patient, so the ambulance took us there. It was trying, having to wait so long.

The doctor had just finished up another surgery, so she wanted a little nap before she started on me. But I felt fine after having taken the painkiller.

Another ultrasound was done. We were told of the dangers of ectopic pregnancies. They also made us aware of the risks during surgery. There could be damage to the bowel, bladder or blood vessels. We were so thankful that no damage was found.

At 8:45 I was wheeled into the operating room, given anesthesia and fell into a peaceful sleep. A small incision was

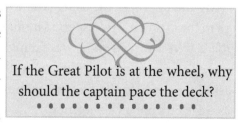

If the Great Pilot is at the wheel, why should the captain pace the deck?

made at my belly button. The pelvis was inspected and the ectopic was noted. It appeared to be unruptured, but nearly at the point of rupturing.

Another incision was made over the area of the ectopic. The clot and pregnancy tissue was removed (or so they thought). There was not much bleeding. I had lost around 200 ccs of blood which was noted in the pelvis, and lost 20 ccs during surgery.

"When she awakes...and feels like going home...she may go..." My anesthesia was wearing off and I was falling asleep and waking up in intervals. I fought to stay awake and tell my husband I want to go home, only to find myself falling into a light sleep again. Finally all was clear and I was fully awake.

At 4:30 p.m. I was released. I was told to take it easy and do no heavy lifting. I was given an appointment for a checkup on February 18th, one and one half weeks later.

I felt great, almost like nothing had happened, never knowing we weren't through yet. The day before my appointment, I was experiencing pain on my right side again. I also had some bleeding and pressure. We called in to Dr. Cant's office and were told to come in right away. I lay on the back seat on the way to the office, trying to relieve the pressure.

It was 2:00 p.m. when we arrived at the doctor's office. After I signed my name, I began to feel faint and sweaty. I quickly sat in a chair till someone brought a wheelchair. My husband pushed me down the aisle to the waiting doctor. I was put on the examining table, and by then I was beginning to feel better again. She pressed on my right side which was only slightly tender, which puzzled her.

I was put in the ambulance again and sent to the hospital for an ultrasound. She said she would meet me there, as something is wrong. I was put on IV.

At the hospital, nurses checked me while waiting on Dr. Cant. I was told I'm unstable, with decreasing blood pressure. My husband went to sign papers and the nurses also left the room. Feeling hot and sweating, I pressed the nurse alarm.

Things happened fast then. The ultrasound was not important anymore. Six or so nurses came and Dr. Cant was giving orders. My dress was cut apart. Two large-bore IVs were placed wide open for fluid resuscitation. They kept talking to me, as they feared I would pass out, but I remained conscious.

Two other doctors were waiting till Dr. Cant came, then I was given anesthesia. Within minutes, I was in the operating room, from 4:10 till 5:15. My blood pressure had improved with the rapid infusion of IV fluids. A four-inch incision was made, lower than the first one. A large amount of blood clots were found in the abdomen. The right tube had ruptured and was bleeding profusely. The tube was clamped to stop the bleeding. Part of the tube was taken out. I had lost about 1,000 ccs of blood.

Waking up went better this time, and I was once more taken to the recovery room. Besides being very weak, I felt great. I ate well and soon felt like going home. Dr. N came in on Friday, the 19th, and since all looked great, I was released. But I had orders to take care and no heavy lifting, with someone to help me out a few days.

For three days I rested a lot, but it seemed I wasn't getting any stronger. Soon I couldn't take the children's noises anymore, so we had them at my husband's parents for a while. My nights seemed long, as sleep wouldn't come. I had no appetite and even water made me nauseous.

One evening my friends were going to town and said they'd bring home anything I was hungry for. Blueberry yogurt appealed to me most, but after taking a spoonful or two I had enough. That night I walked the floor or looked at books to pass the time. I wasn't really sick, yet something was wrong, as I felt really weak. I was overjoyed to see the neighbor's lights go on around 4:30. This awful night had finally come to an end, and my dear husband would soon be awake.

Five o' clock found us at the hospital again. I was dehydrated, so I was put on IV for awhile. Within an hour, I felt like a totally new person that could laugh again. I felt much stronger, although I was a bit short of breath from low blood count.

We asked the doctor what I could have done differently, as I had been drinking lots of water. We were told that sodas or juice with a lot of sugar would have prevented dehydration. Also being up and around more would have increased my appetite.

I recovered quickly after that. We thank the Lord for sparing my life. We really learned a lot in that short month. Our doctors and nurses were very kind and took time off to visit with us. Dr. Cant said it's extremely rare that the first laser surgery does not work.

Two or three of my nurses told me they had experienced a tubal and became pregnant three to five months later. At first I thought, *Not me*. But as time went on, God had other plans. In June I was pregnant once more. We got an ultrasound done to make sure all is well. On August 4, 1999, the ultrasound showed a little girl and all appeared fine. On March 19, 2000, our precious little girlie was born with no difficulties. Later we were blessed with three more little ones.

The following poem became special to me:

The Love of God

God is love; His mercy brightens
All the path in which we move;
Bliss He forms, and woe He lightens;
God is light, and God is love.

Chance and change are busy ever;
Worlds decay, and ages move;
But His mercy waneth never
God is light, and God is love.

E'en the hour that darkest seemeth
Will His changeless goodness prove,
From the mist His brightness streameth;
God is light, and God is love.

He with earthly cares entwineth
Hope and comfort from above;
Everywhere His glory shineth;
God is light, and God is love.

Art thou weary, tender heart?
Be glad of pain.
In sorrow sweetest things will grow,
As flowers in the rain.
Be patient! Thou wilt have the sun
When clouds their perfect work have done.

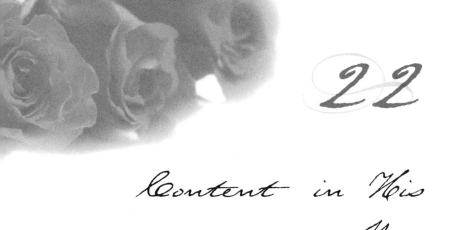

22

Content in His Will

—anonymous

WE HAD TWO healthy children, ages one and three years old. They were totally normal pregnancies. Then in September of 2003 I was one week late with my period, so I started wondering if I might be pregnant again.

On Monday (when my period was one week late), I had just a little cramping and some spotting. I thought I might be starting with a late period. By Wednesday, I still hadn't started with my period, so I called my doctor. She advised me to get a pregnancy test at the store. We had plans on going shopping Friday evening, so I decided I would get one then. (Since we are Amish, it wasn't so easy to drive to the store and purchase one.)

Tuesday and Wednesday mornings when I got out of bed, I had some pain in my lower left side, but it seemed to ease up by lunchtime. On Wednesday evening I was in the garden pulling out green bean plants. That night I had some more spotting. Earlier it had been medium to dark brown spotting, but now it was bright red.

On Thursday morning at 3:00 I woke up with what seemed

to be a very painful period, so I took Tylenol. I'd always experienced painful cramps during periods, even as a girl, so it didn't seem unusual.

Ten minutes later I threw up and had severe stomach pain. It seemed to be worse on my lower left side. I lay down on the living room floor, hoping to get relief. My husband stayed home from work that morning.

Around 7:00 I wanted to get up from the floor. I got to my hands and knees, but it hurt so bad that I couldn't stand up. (I wonder if this is when the tube burst.) I was so miserable. I had tremendous pressure in my rectal area when I went to the toilet. I also had loose, dark stools.

At 8:00 my husband called the doctor, but he happened to be out of town. They gave us the phone number of her backup doctor. By then I was so weak and light-headed I had to sit on the edge of the bathtub to fix my hair. My pain wasn't so sharp anymore, but I hurt all over my abdomen and up to my shoulders.

On the way to the doctor, I hunched over a big pillow to make the ride bearable. When we walked into the doctor's waiting room, the lady at the desk handed us a clipboard with three papers to sign. I signed my name and told my husband I have to lie down or I'll pass out. So a nurse took me to a room and had me lie on the examining table. My shoulders hurt almost as much as my abdomen and I was shaking all over.

The doctor asked some questions, such as how many days late my period was, etc. She then inserted a needle into my vagina and drew out blood. This made her sure I had a tubal. She called for a wheelchair, and a nurse pushed me over to the hospital, right beside the doctor's office.

I realized how serious this really was when the doctor ran ahead of me to change into operating clothes. In about ten minutes I was on the operating table.

When I got out of surgery, I was very weak and rundown. My left tube had burst, so she removed it, in addition to a cyst on my right tube. I had lost one and a half liters of blood and was given two units.

On Saturday when I came home, I was emotionally and physically drained. I tried not to wonder, "Why me?" too much because I needed all my strength to get my health back. We got a hired girl to do the housework and take care of our two children. I was awfully sore, even though I only had three small incisions.

I found Proverbs 3:5,6 very comforting. "Trust in the Lord with all thine heart, and lean not unto thine own understanding. In all thy ways acknowledge him, and he shall direct thy paths."

Six weeks after the operation I had a checkup. I was healing okay. The doctor was good at answering my many questions. She said I might never again have a tubal, and yet there's a good chance of it happening again. She said it's very important that I come into the office when my period is late, so they can determine where the pregnancy is. She made sure I understood that if this happens on my other side, then I couldn't have any more children. If they can detect a tubal before the tube ruptures, they can save the tube but not the pregnancy .

Six months after my tubal, I became pregnant again. I had some unusual cramping and spotting. The doctor did an ultrasound, which showed excess blood in the uterus. She did exploratory surgery to make sure it's not in my other tube. This time she made two incisions. Thankfully it was not in my tube. But, unfortunately, two weeks later I miscarried. My spirits were pretty low this time. My doctor told me miscarriages happen all the time, and since we have two healthy children, we had a good chance of having more.

In April of 2006 we were blessed with a precious baby boy, but not without complications. First I had a blood clot in my uterus that caused some nerve-racking spotting. Then I had placenta previa which straightened up toward the end of my pregnancy.

We are so thankful to the Lord for allowing us this precious bundle. I can not help but think we will never have a large family after all my body has gone through already. But I want to be content in the Lord's will, and leave it in His hands.

Be strong and of a good courage; be not afraid, neither be thou dismayed: for the Lord thy God is with thee whithersoever thou goest. Joshua 1:9

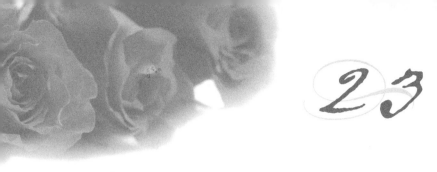

23

God's Healing Touch

—*John & Miriam Miller, Millersburg, OH*

THANK GOD WE serve a Mighty Physician! We have just had an experience that we will never forget. I thought I was pregnant because I had missed my period. At five weeks along I got sick. I kept passing out and had pain on my left side, besides vomiting, etc. At that time we thought it might be the flu.

We did two pregnancy tests, but both showed negative. Then I noticed the information in the box where it said a tubal pregnancy may show negative. Since the HCG level is not as high as in a normal pregnancy, it doesn't always pick it up.

I looked up the symptoms of tubals and it was exactly what I was experiencing. At six weeks I started bleeding, so we thought it might be a miscarriage. But then my pain started getting more severe and I kept doubling over in pain, passing out, having headaches and severe shoulder and neck pain. My bleeding stayed at a minimum if I was in bed, but if I'd get up it would just gush out.

Finally, on Monday, February 19, 2007, we knew we had to do something. The midwife told us there is nothing natural that they know of to do for a tubal and explained to us the seriousness of it.

We called our pastor and he told us they and the saints all

over the states are lifting me up to the throne of God. We should also pray about it and ask the Lord to show us what we should do.

My husband tried calling two of our former doctors. The first one wasn't there and the second one was too busy to talk. The staff told us we can't talk to the doctor now, but they could make an appointment for us to see him the next day. My dear husband tried to explain to them how serious it is and that we needed to see the doctor right away. They didn't seem to know anything about tubals. So I told my husband to just hang up since they didn't know anything about it. I knew Someone else whom we could talk to 24 hours a day, Who knows a whole lot more than all the doctors put together.

We prayed and wept together and trusted in the Lord for whatever He had for us. Two hours later He miraculously touched my body, and I had no more pain. It took a few minutes to fully comprehend what had actually happened. I wondered if my pain left, only to come back again?

But praise to God, it was really true! I was still very weak from all that I'd gone through. Then three days later I had a blood clot in my left leg, so I was bedridden again. But I praise God for all this. I know I have come through, trusting more and having my faith strengthened.

So was it a tubal or what? Only our Good Lord knows. All we know is I had all the symptoms of it. I can never fully explain the peace I had those last two hours before my pain left. Oh, to think of entering into Heaven to be with Jesus forevermore! You might say, "Didn't you think of your husband and children?" Yes, but I knew God would be able to take better care of them than I could.

Sometimes we forget so easily what we are here on earth for. I think it would be good for everyone to come face to face with death. You might think this sounds depressing. Really, it's not, if we're right with God!

These earthly, material things have so little meaning. We're not promised tomorrow. May the Lord bless and strengthen whoever is going through a difficult situation. Always remember, the Lord is available 24 hours a day!

Editor's note: It is my belief that an embryo may have worked itself out of the tube. This happens in rare occasions where the embryo is close to the end of the tube. But remember, this will not work for everyone! In the majority of situations, the doctors need to do their part too. Prayer alone will not save your life in some cases.

> When the train goes through a tunnel and the world gets dark, do you jump out? Of course not. You sit still and trust the engineer to get you through.
> —Corrie Ten Boom

A TEAR FROM MY HEART

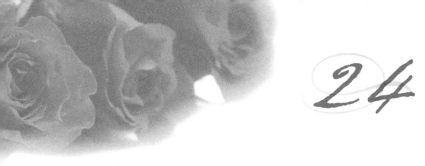

24

Emotional Seesaws

—J. Edward & Ella Weaver, Stanley, NY

IT WAS EARLY in the morning in April of 1995, after Edward went out to the barn to start with the chores, that I first knew something was wrong. I had a cold and was coughing pretty hard when I had this sharp pain in my abdomen. I assumed I just stretched something from coughing so much, so I went out to the barn to milk cows as usual while Edward did the feeding.

I never did get the milking done, as my pain was just too severe. I lay on some hay bales while Edward did the chores. Every so often he came to check on me and ask if I'm okay.

Since we knew I was pregnant, it was in the back of our minds that it could be an ectopic, but it was something so uncommon that we thought, "Surely not." We thought of gallstone attacks or appendicitis and hoped that it was one of these.

We waited until the doctor's office hours before calling. We put the children to the neighbors after they had breakfast. It really would have been wiser to go to the emergency room right away.

At the doctor's office I got severe pain in my upper back and didn't feel the other pain anymore. The doctor said that's a sign of internal bleeding. He suspected an ectopic and called the hospital to tell them we're coming. But they seemed so slow to us. While answering questions I passed out, which made them hurry more.

When I got back from surgery, they told me they had tried laser, but since it was too severe, they needed to make bigger incisions. They felt I had lost about three pints of blood, and gave me one unit. I was really weak and needed to stay four days. I also had pneumonia, which we felt was probably from my cold, even though it could have come from surgery.

Since I was totally breast-feeding our baby at nine months, and she hardly accepted anything else, Edward brought her along in when he came to visit each day. I was glad I could continue nursing.

We were thankful for the help we had with the chores and children. Grandmother took our two-year-old along home, and he had his second birthday while there. It was hard to let him go to Pennsylvania, but we knew it would be a while till I'd be able to do my motherly duties again.

Our oldest boys were three and four years old. It had looked quite overwhelming at times to think of having another little one, even though I had always thought I'd like to have a big family.

We did fear it might happen again, especially the first few years after my ectopic. But then it happened numerous times that we lost our babies at two to four months, and I always needed a D&C. So we have been on an emotional seesaw over the years. It always affected me more emotionally than physically. We are glad for good health, even if this is not as we would have chosen.

I often pondered on the verses: "Ask, and it shall be given you...whatsoever ye shall ask, I will give you," and "Delight thyself also in the Lord, and he shall give thee the desires of thine heart."

We must remember that our spiritual health is most important, so what we might wish for might not be best for us, and we might receive leanness unto our soul in receiving our wishes. And we are to delight ourselves in the Lord and then our desires are however He sees best.

Life might seem long and we feel deprived of a large family as wished for, but really, all of this shall pass away in a short time. We want to enjoy the blessings that God has so freely bestowed upon us. As we fill our lives with worthwhile things, and think of others in their trials, we will find life fullfilling. Since we are human, we will not be without struggles. With God all things are possible. We appreciated all the understanding friends along life's journey.

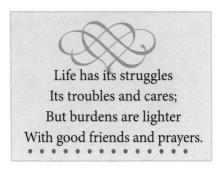

Life has its struggles
Its troubles and cares;
But burdens are lighter
With good friends and prayers.

A TEAR FROM MY HEART

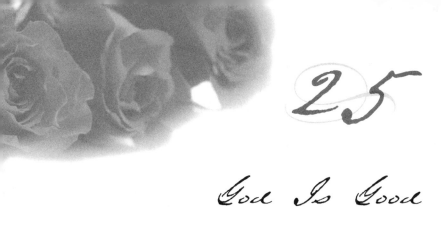

25

God Is Good

—Randy & Wilma Lapp, Kenya, East Africa

IT WAS MAY 1998 in Gap, PA. I was delighted to be pregnant again. Krystal, our firstborn, was eleven months old, and it was a dream of ours to have the two oldest close together in age.

However, a few weeks after I missed my period, I started spotting. I blamed the spotting on a fall I had the day before while cleaning windows.

I called my faithful midwife and she gave me lots of advice, including various herbs to take to prevent a miscarriage. I rested, propped up my feet and read. The spotting continued, but I thought it was very strange that I did not miscarry.

My husband and I planted sweet corn one evening. If I would have been listening to my body, I would have admitted something seems strange. I was tired and feeling a pain that would not go away. I read the book *What to Expect When You're Expecting* and noticed what it said about a tubal pregnancy. I was scared when I realized I had almost all of those symptoms.

I called my midwife and she promised to come to our house. I fainted over lunch time. The severe pain caused me to toss and turn in bed, making it impossible to relax.

The midwife came by later that afternoon, and pushed

down on my abdomen. When she released, I felt pain. She concluded I have the feared—a tubal. I shed tears. She prayed with us before Randy and I left for the hosptial. God gave me peace in the midst of a storm.

The ultrasound once again confirmed the tubal pregnancy. While being wheeled into surgery, I was extremely uncomfortable, but I tried to be brave. Alas, the doctor was not there. He had another emergency call. It seemed like I was waiting an hour in that cold, bright room, while the nurses explained in detail what insrtuments would be used during surgery.

Pain, oh, what pain after the surgery, and the distressing news that the tube had to be removed. The tube had already burst, but infection had not spread to the rest of the system, because it had been blocked off. I give God the glory first of all, and also the herbs I had taken to prevent a miscarriage.

I arrived home from the hospital in severe pain—so much pain that I wanted to die. I was not hungry until the next day when my mother toasted and buttered a piece of bread and poured some boiling water over it.

I felt five years older. I wrote out many prayers to the Lord. The book of Psalms brought comfort to my hurting heart. Isaiah 41:10 continued to be one of my favorite Bible verses.

Many were the days that I wondered if Krystal will be an only child, especially after my miscarriage in 1999. It was a tough time for my husband and me. My midwife once again assisted in herbs, encouragement and love.

In January of 2000, Ryan was born. He was an answer to prayer, such a delight and joy to us all. Eighteen months later, in July of 2001, Tyler was born. Indeed a blessing!

We are in Kenya, East Africa, as missionaries since April 2004. Our third son, Matthew, was born in December 2005, after a miscarriage in September 2004.

God is good. These precious lives are gifts from above. We praise God for His strength and peace at all times. Praise God for answered prayers. God is good!

Looking ahead, it's a mountain of days
Through which you have to climb.
But they become only little hills
When taken one day at a time.

Answered Prayer

My Lord, sometimes I wonder
If you still hear my prayer,
If you will never answer,
If you no longer care.
My faith begins to falter;
I feel depressed and blue;
I cry out my frustration
And disappointment, too.

Then, suddenly and clearly,
An answer, Lord, you show:
Your Word reveals so plainly
The way that I should go.
From unexpected sources
Your aid supplies my need;
My harsh conditions lighten;
My fettered wings are freed.

How surely, Lord, you show me
That still you truly care;
You know my every burden;
You hear my every prayer.
You have a time, a purpose,
A reason for each test;
Your love so great, you give me
Just what You know is best.

I thank You, Lord! I thank You
For answering my cry,
For showing that Your Presence
Is ever standing by,
That Your forgiveness covers
My doubts, my sadness too.
How can I fully offer
My thanks, O Lord, to You?

Mrs. Silas Bowman

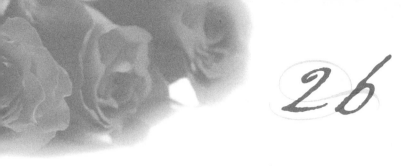

26

The Story of My Tubal Pregnancy

—*anonymous*

I HAD NOT known I was pregnant. My first sign of something unusual going on was the start of an early period. It was ten days early. I wondered what's going on, as I had been on a regular schedule for a while already since our last baby. But since my toddler was still nursing frequently, I figured that might have something to do with it, so I didn't worry about it.

Still, it just did not seem like a period. It had dark spotting every day for a week, and it still hadn't stopped. I started thinking about a miscarriage and asked a friend who had experience in that line. But she didn't think it sounded like a miscarriage.

I thought of calling my midwife, but I felt fine and wasn't having any pain at all. I decided it must be just a weird period.

Finally, after twelve days of spotting, it stopped. By then it rather bothered me that I had put up with it so long and hadn't called my midwife. But it had stopped now, and I felt fine, so why worry about it now?

No other problem showed up until exactly a week after the spotting had ended. I started with stomach pains in the afternoon. It reminded me of how I sometimes felt during ovulation, so I assumed that's what it is. But I soon decided my pain is a lot worse than I ever experienced during ovulation.

I was able to keep on working, and by supper time I felt better again. Later in the evening the pain got a lot worse, though. It hurt to walk or sit so I lay down. It also hurt to lie on my side or back, but when I lay flat on my stomach I was able to bear it. I got the chills, first hot, then cold.

I really wondered what's wrong with me, as I had never felt like this before. It never once entered my mind that it could be something life-threatening. By bedtime I felt better, so we went to bed and slept, completely unaware of what was going on inside my body. God's protecting hand was over us. Instead of bleeding to death, my blood clotted and slowed down. (This is when we think it ruptured.)

By morning I felt much better, but walking and sitting still bothered me somewhat. I started spotting again, so I thought, "Oh, that's why I was so sick yesterday. I'm starting with another early period."

Four days after my tube had ruptured, I started having pains again. When I lay flat on my stomach I was able to bear it. I felt worse this time, faintish and nauseated. (My doctor informed us later that this time my body was reacting to all the junk it was receiving—blood and clots.) I was also having loose, painful bowel movements ever since my tube had ruptured. Now they got even worse. I thought I could hardly bear the

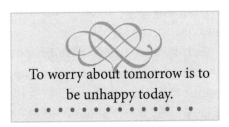

To worry about tomorrow is to be unhappy today.

pain.

In the following days I kept thinking I should contact the midwife, but each day I pushed it off till the next day, sure that it will go away again. I was able to keep on with my work, but I just didn't feel right and had these unbearable bowel movements.

Finally, a week after my tube had ruptured, I decided, "This is not normal, and it's not getting any better." So I called my midwife and told her I'm having a problem with my periods. I'm getting them too often, they're lasting too long and twice I got very sick.

She gave me some suggestions, but also said that's how tubals work. She asked me to do a pregnancy test. I did one right away and it showed positive. I thought it couldn't be! All these problems I'd been putting up with the last four weeks, and here I was pregnant, and not even doing anything about it.

It was six weeks since my last normal period. The midwife informed us that if it is a tubal and at six weeks pregnant, there is no time to lose. She sent us for an ultrasound right away. Since the tube had already ruptured, they could not find it on the ultrasound. They said it could be a miscarriage or a cyst that caused the pain.

I had never been in a hospital before. I just couldn't believe this was happening to me. Why me? I had never had problems before. Always it had been other people.

Not until four ultrasounds and four trips to the hospital, did they decide to do surgery. They still weren't sure what they would find, but suspected a tube that had ruptured when I first experienced pain.

During my last two days at home before the surgery, I started feeling very weak and light-headed. I was also losing weight fast. I lost approximately 15 pounds.

My surgery was eight days after the first ultrasound and two and one half weeks after my tube had ruptured. My blood had formed a large clot, but I had been bleeding some daily and getting low in blood, which explained the weak feeling.

Placental tissue had grown fast to my appendix, ovary, bladder and large blood vessel. So in addition to removing the tube, I also had the appendix and ovary removed. Since it was life-threatening, I had a three-day hospital stay.

The future is unknown. We long for a bigger family, and yet the idea of getting pregnant again looks scary.

I hope by writing my story, it will help other women discover their problem sooner. If I had known tubals act like this, I would have taken action right away, when I first started with an early unusual period.

Casting all your care upon him; for he careth for you. I Peter 5:7

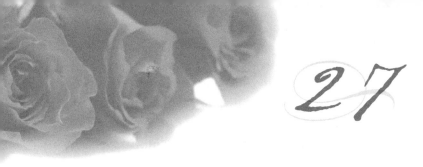

27

Shared Struggles
The Mother's Story

—*Pauline Frey, Drayton, ON*

THE DAY OF May 30, 1998, started out as another ordinary day with Darrell going to work at Maco Enterprises. I got breakfast for our children, Patrick, age 3, Philip, 22 months, and Veronica, 6 months. In the morning I baby-sat our neighbor's daughter while she went shopping. It was close to dinner time when she came back, so I asked her to stay since I had more food left over than what the children and I could eat. As we were washing dishes I asked her how long a period should last. I had show for over a week since my regular flow. This was unusual for me. I wasn't sure how soon you should be concerned and see a doctor about something like this.

After supper we put the children to bed at the usual time. As Darrell and I were getting ready for bed a sharp pain hit my lower abdomen. It didn't last long, but I had an uneasy feeling and an ache that made us decide to go to the hospital. We called Darrell's mom to stay with the children while we get it checked out.

At the hospital the nurse asked questions and took a pregnancy test, which showed positive. Since it's a small hospital, she needed to call a doctor in to see me. The doctor

A TEAR FROM MY HEART 163

told the nurse that it sounds like it is the start of a miscarriage. He didn't come in to see me, but told her to tell us to come back in the morning to see our own doctor. I felt uneasy to go home since a miscarriage sounded scary. The nurse thought I would sleep better in my own bed and that a miscarriage isn't something that can't be handled at home. I found it hard to believe I was pregnant. We had a six-month-old baby.

When we got home Mom said that she could come back in the morning to keep the children when Darrell and I go to the hospital again. I was surprised that I slept very well.

The next morning I wanted a drink of water, but I couldn't get up. Darrell tried to help me sit up, but I had sharp pain. I decided I wasn't that thirsty and left it at that. Darrell wanted to go to work to organize the day, since he is the manager there. When his mom came, he left.

Mom got the children dressed and gave them their breakfast. I asked her for a drink, but the same thing happened. I was gasping for breath. Mom was sure this was something unusual. She called Darrell and said she thinks we should go to the hospital right away.

After Darrell was dressed, he tried to help me get up, but I couldn't. He decided to call the ambulance. It took awhile to get there, and we found out from others later that you need to make it sound really serious if you want them to come fast. Mom had the children wave to me by the window, but I didn't see them. We drove away without sirens going and flashers flashing. I really wondered what was wrong. Did the nurse know what she was talking about the evening before? I had a lot of pain when I moved and yet they didn't hurry.

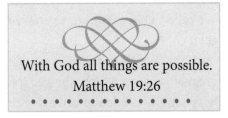

With God all things are possible.
Matthew 19:26

The ambulance attendance left me with a nurse at the hospital. Soon our family doctor came in. I gave him the report that I found out the evening before. He wanted me to lie on my back. Since I couldn't breathe and needed to gasp for breath, he put me on oxygen.

Darrell understood the doctor saying something to the nurse about ordering three units of blood. They were hurrying around like it was an emergency. Still I didn't know what was wrong. I had never heard about a ruptured tubal pregnancy.

Another nurse came in with a portable ultrasound machine. Since the hospital is small, they have a surgeon in on certain days of the week. Thankfully this was the day he was in. He came bounding in. He took one look at the ultrasound saying something about my tube and surgery. Poor people that were booked for surgery had to wait; this was an emergency.

They had me on a cot and were wheeling me away before Darrell or I knew what was happening. I never had surgery before, so I didn't have much time to think what it all means.

I remember the nurse in the operating room taking out my hair pins. I tried telling her I didn't want to be lying on my back. It hurt so much. Soon I saw a doctor putting a mask over my face. I recognized this doctor. He was the doctor on call from the evening before. I wonder what he thought. I would have been saved from losing all the blood I did if they would have caught it sooner. I forgave him. They have many cases that don't end like mine did.

The next thing I knew I was with Darrell in the recovery room. A nurse came and checked up on us, too. I was on IV for blood transfusions and on painkiller. Later in the afternoon I was put in a hospital room. I had two blood transfusions given instead of three like the doctor had been talking about. They did not have laser to work with here at this hospital. so the recovery was like someone who has a cesarean.

I asked Darrell what the problem was that I had surgery. He answered the questions as best as he knew. I could understand better why I had so much pain after I realized how much internal bleeding there had been. The doctor thought I was maybe four to six weeks pregnant, since this is when it usually makes a problem.

I was really tired the first few days. On the third day they gave me liquids to drink and by the next day I could eat. I had the IV removed on the fourth day. I had family and some friends visit me, which helped the time go faster. I had time to think what all had happened. I was glad I wasn't pregnant anymore. I thought I had enough work with the three children we had. God in His love took care of this in a different way than I imagined it would happen to us. Some people asked if I believe that our baby is in Heaven. I never really knew I was pregnant so I did not really think much about this, until people asked me how I felt about it.

Since Veronica was only six months old I wasn't supposed to lift her up. Some kind girls from our youth helped us out for four weeks. After that I had help one day a week for the busy times in the summer.

Since this happening in '98 we have been blessed with four more children. Being with only one tube didn't take away children from us. Eighteen months after this happening we had another daughter born to us. It would have been a disappointment to us if we wouldn't have had any more children.

God is love, His mercy brightens
All the paths in which we move.
Bliss He forms and woe He lightens,
God is light, and God is love.

The Father's Story

—*Darrell Frey, Drayton, ON*

MY OWN MEMORIES of Pauline's experience over eight years ago have faded somewhat, but I will still attempt to get together what I remember. Although I'm sure Pauline told me about her abnormal conditions, I don't specifically remember it. We were getting ready for bed when she experienced a very sharp pain. After waiting for a while with no apparent change, we decided to at least call the hospital and talk to a nurse. After explaining the symptoms, she advised us to come up and get it checked out. I called my mom, and she very willingly agreed to stay with our children while we were gone.

After our arrival at Palmerston Hospital, a twenty-minute drive away, the nurses soon determined that my wife was pregnant. This was a surprise to us, but that still did not explain what the pain was all about. The nurse suggested that it could be a miscarriage. After discussing this on the phone with the on-call doctor, she recommended we go home for the night, then come back at nine the next morning to see the doctor. We took the nurse's advice and went home again.

Surprisingly, Pauline had a relatively good night and slept reasonably well. My mom came again the next morning so I could go to the shop and organize the employees' work for the day. I planned to stay until it was time to take Pauline to the hospital, but I wasn't at work very long until Mom called me and said that Pauline has extreme pain, and she thinks I should take her up to the hospital right away.

When I entered our bedroom, she was lying on her left side with her back towards me. When I asked her to try and get up to go out to the car, she moved a little, then moaned and said she cannot. With such a reaction, the hospital suddenly seemed far away. I asked Pauline what she wants me to do, and the quick reply was, "Better call an ambulance." I made the call, got changed and threw some clothes in a bag for Pauline. After about twenty minutes, the ambulance finally arrived, and soon they had Pauline on a stretcher and wheeled her out to the ambulance. The paramedics suggested that I drive to the hospital myself, so that I have a vehicle there. I asked my mom to call Pauline's parents and also Linda, our neighbors across the road from us, then hurried to the hospital.

When I arrived at the hospital, I had to wait a little until a nurse took me in to the examination room where Pauline was lying on a bed. Our family doctor came in very soon. He asked some questions about her condition, then asked her to lie on her back. I remember watching him do the examination and pressing on her abdomen. "Does this hurt?" "Does this hurt?" Other than these questions, he did not say anything and I really wondered what he was thinking. This was extremely painful for Pauline, so she was quite relieved when he was done with the examination. I was asked what her blood type is, and the doctor asked a nurse to get three units of blood. At this point I was still rather naive about the whole situation. Three units of blood did not seem like a significant amount of blood to me, until later, when I learned that people only have about 5 L of blood in their body.

The doctor asked for an ultrasound, and to get an IV started. While he was waiting, he tried to insert a needle into Pauline's wrist for an IV. He slapped her wrists and tried again, but was unsuccessful. He did this a few more times, but finally gave up and asked a nurse to try. She was able to get it started. I thought perhaps it was something the doctor did not do very often, but found out later that since Pauline had lost a lot of blood, her veins had started to collapse which made it very difficult to insert a needle.

A technician came in with the ultrasound machine, then our family doctor watched for a little, then left the room with Pauline, and I was still wondering what her problem was. A few minutes later an older, dark-skinned man dressed in hospital scrubs, with paper slippers, came shuffling in. He walked up to the ultrasound monitor and watched as the technician maneuvered the wand around on Pauline's abdomen. After watching the ultrasound for a little, the man who I thought might be a janitor pointed to a spot on the monitor and asked, "What's that thing?" The technician and the nurses laughed at his question, and then he shuffled out again, with the sound of his paper footwear fading down the hallway. A few minutes later our family doctor came in, and he was

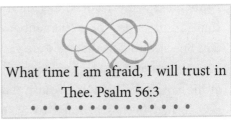

What time I am afraid, I will trust in Thee. Psalm 56:3

ready to talk. He explained that Pauline has a ruptured tubal pregnancy, and they would need to do surgery as soon as possible since she was having internal bleeding. He said this is what he suspected, but he wanted the surgeon to confirm it. It was then that I discovered the person who I had guessed to be a janitor was the surgeon!

Our family doctor told me that I can go to the waiting room, then someone would let me know when the surgery was over. I used the pay phone there to call my mom and Pauline's parents to tell them what's happening. My mother-in-law responded by saying that we need to leave it in the hands of the Lord. After about a forty-five-minute wait, the family doctor came to the waiting room. He told me to come back to the nurses' station with him. There he explained that the surgery was done and had been successful. They removed her tube, and he said that he guessed she had lost about 2500 ccs (2.5 L) of blood. He apologized that they had to remove her tube, but then added that at least I still have my wife. I realized that he did not say this only to make me feel good, but because it was the truth! After this statement sunk into my numb mind, the seriousness of this whole experience finally dawned on me. If nothing would have been done, Pauline would have bled to death. Truly God is to be praised!

I spent the next few hours in the recovery room with Pauline, giving her ice chips and discussing her experience. Later she was moved into a hospital room. When we discussed the day's happenings with a nurse, she mentioned that Pauline had caused a great deal of excitement at their small hospital that day. She also told us that we were very fortunate to be able to have the surgery done within forty-five minutes after arriving at the hospital. This was because that morning a number of people had been scheduled to have minor surgeries done there. For this reason they had a surgeon at the hospital, as well as an anesthesiologist, and our family doctor who was at the hospital when Pauline came. If any of these three would not have been present, it would have delayed surgery.

On my way home that day, I stopped in to tell Linda about Pauline's experience, since my mom had not been able to get hold of Linda. She had been at home most of the day, but their telephone was not working so we were unable to call her. She was quite surprised to hear about our experiences of the day. She said that she had met the ambulance on her way back from town that morning, but did not realize that it was her neighbor who was in it.

After a few days Pauline was allowed to come home, but

was not allowed to do any lifting because of the danger of the incision reopening. Pauline's mom called around and found someone who was able to help Pauline with the housework for a few weeks. Pauline had help for about four weeks, then after that we were on our own again.

The doctor told Pauline that her chance of conceiving is lower with only one tube left, but it is still possible to have more children. In the eight years after this experience, God blessed us with four more children—one boy and three more girls.

The rocky road before you may lead
to a rainbow.

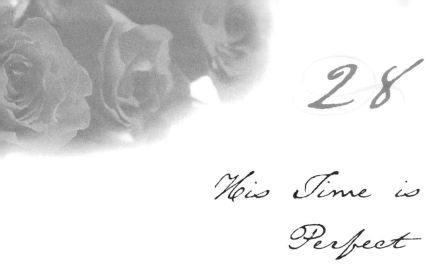

28

His Time is Perfect

—Alan & Mary Priest, Burns Lake, BC

IN MARCH OF 1981, the time of my tubal pregnancy, I was a busy mother with three little girls. The oldest was two years, nine months, the second was one year, nine months, and the baby was six months old.

We lived a distance from church, and Alan, my husband, had a meeting prior to prayer meeting on this particular day. The girls and I went along and stayed with my sister and family until the service. During that time, I started to have pain in my abdomen. It was more comfortable to bend and lean on the kitchen counter than to stand up straight.

"Just a stomachache," we thought, and went to prayer meeting. It was hard to hold a wiggly baby with the pain I was having, and I could hardly wait to get home and put the babies to bed.

When that was finally done, I went to bed and tried to get into a comfortable position to sleep. I dozed awhile, then the pain woke me up, so I got up and moved around to see if it would let up. Eventually, the pressure let up, but bleeding immediately started. We had no idea what was wrong, but assumed it was an irregular menstrual period.

For the next four days, I did not feel well, and the flow continued. I dragged myself through the necessary work and care of the children, even hosting the visiting minister and his family on Sunday.

Finally, on Tuesday morning, the sixth day after the pain started, I awoke with such pain that it was hard to move around and care for the family. Alan gave the girls breakfast and made a doctor appointment for me.

We live in a long way from town, and have to cross a lake by ferry to get there. On the way to the ferry, we had a flat tire. My pain was relentless, and I prayed we would not miss the ferry and have to wait another hour. We did not miss it, and kept the appointment, by God's help.

The doctor concluded that I had a tubal pregnancy and that my tube had burst that night after prayer meeting, nearly a week before, when the bleeding started.

From where I was in my cycle, I couldn't believe I was pregnant, and I never have understood that part of it.

We had left our baby with Alan's parents at home, but had taken the one- and two-year-olds along to town. Alan took them to friends, and came to be with me at the hospital. Surgery was scheduled for 7:00 that evening, March 31, 1981. I felt so terrible that I was willing to undergo whatever it took to get rid of the pain. It felt like a giant cramp that would not let go.

My husband had to pick up the girls and get the last ferry of the evening, but he stayed till I woke up. Of course, I felt groggy and sore, but things were on the mend.

When the nurses bustled in the next morning, they said, "We thought Dr. Magee was pulling a joke on us when he told us to prepare for your surgery last evening."

My doctor told me, "Your abdomen was full of blood, which had to be cleaned out. That made the procedure take longer. The blood can also paralyze the organs, so it might take awhile until the bowels work properly." I think it was unusual for anyone to go so long with a burst tube.

From then on, it was an effort of patience until the IV was removed, until a fever and chills episode was remedied, and my eating and digestion could resume.

It would not have been wise to go home too soon, because we lived so far from the hospital, where the care was good and quite personal, because it was a small hospital. But finally, on the sixth day, my doctor released me. What a joy to go home to my family!

We have been very thankful that God watched over us in what could have been a life-threatening situation, although we did not recognize it as such.

We have also been thankful that God gave us four more children after the surgery. They are all grown up now. We still live in the same area that is reached by a ferry across Francois Lake in central British Columbia.

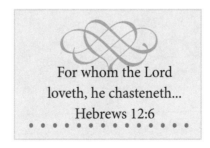

For whom the Lord
loveth, he chasteneth...
Hebrews 12:6

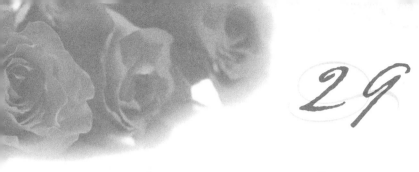

29

God is in Control

WE WERE MARRIED for a half year when I decided I might be pregnant. My period was a week late and I was used to getting it right on time.

One Saturday morning I woke up with terrible pain in my left side. I was doubled over with pain, so I couldn't do much. By about 2:00 p.m. it got better. I didn't know what it was. I thought it might be a stomach virus, as my husband had it a few days before. For some reason the idea that I might be pregnant wasn't even considered. I had been helping my husband dig and pull out some shrubs the evening before and thought I could possibly have strained a muscle. We didn't think too much about this and put it behind us.

The next day I wasn't feeling like myself yet, and that evening I started bleeding, just a little brownish spotting. We thought my period must be starting.

The following morning I had no sign of my period, and the next days I had only some spotting. I decided that either my period is wacky or I'm pregnant and bleeding a little. I knew some women do and everything turns out okay.

On Thursday I told my mom about it, and she told me to do a pregnancy test. If it showed positive, I should call a midwife.

A TEAR FROM MY HEART 177

It showed positive, so I called a midwife. She asked me several questions, and gave me orders to come in as soon as possible. So we went to her office and she checked me out. Yes, I was pregnant and my uterus was enlarged, but why the blood? Was my pain on Saturday connected with this? She decided it must be one of three things: a strained muscle, a miscarriage about to happen or a tubal pregnancy. The first one we both doubted (but would've wanted to believe it), because she commented on my strong stomach muscles and I was used to working hard. We had a blood test done to see if my HCG level was going up the way it does in a normal pregnancy. In the meantime, I was only allowed to make light meals, etc.

On Monday we did a second blood test and talked about an ultrasound. But the midwife was uncertain if it would be worth our money, as it is unlikely that they could see anything at seven weeks. Still, we decided we could at least try. We (especially me) were so tired of not knowing what's wrong. It was very stressful. I was still bleeding, even clots sometimes, but never heavily.

The next day (Tuesday) we did an ultrasound. I was so anxious. What would they find? Of course by now I desperately wanted everything to be okay. Suddenly my pregnancy was very real and I wanted the baby so very badly, but at the same time I wanted out of this dark suspense to know what (if anything) was wrong. I knew God was in control and would work everything out for our good, but of course, I wanted answers.

The ultrasound showed that there was no embryo in my uterus. So we went home and waited to hear from our midwife, who was trying to schedule an appointment for surgery.

Later that evening we found out that surgery might not even

be necessary, as my second blood test showed my HCG level was down to "almost not pregnant." That meant my body was taking care of it, absorbing it, fighting it off the way it would for a cold, etc. Oh, what a relief! Now it seemed our troubles were about over. Yes, we were sad about the loss, but relieved at not having to do surgery.

But we were far from it. The next day my midwife stopped by and told me to sit down; she has something to tell me. She told me that my third blood test (which I had done on Wednesday) showed my level up, further up than my first one had been. The only thing they could figure out was that the second one was a mistake. She called the laboratory and asked them to rerun the second one.

To say the least, it was a huge letdown. It felt like we were on a real roller coaster ride. The midwife made an appointment with the surgeon for Monday morning, to have him give his opinion.

That weekend we spent trying to prepare for what might be ahead of us. I was pretty scared and tried to brace up. We copied some verses from the Bible on a sheet of paper that I carried in my pocket for days.

"My grace is sufficient for thee; for my strength is made perfect in weakness. Most gladly therefore will I rather glory in my infirmities, that the power of Christ may rest upon me. Therefore I take pleasure in infirmities, in reproaches, in necessities, in persecutions, in distresses for Christ's sake: for when I am weak, then am I strong" (II Corinthians 12:9 & 10).

"Be content with such things as ye have: for he hath said, I will never leave thee nor forsake thee. The Lord is my helper, and I will not fear what man shall do unto me" (Hebrews 13:5 & 6).

"Fear thou not; for I am with thee. Be not dismayed; for I am thy God. I will strengthen thee; yea, I will help thee; yea, I will uphold thee with the right hand of my righteousness" (Isaiah 41:10).

"Thou wilt keep him in perfect peace, whose mind is stayed on thee, because he trusteth in thee. Trust ye in the Lord forever: for in the Lord is everlasting strength" (Isaiah 26:3 & 4).

"But even the very hairs of your head are all numbered. Fear not therefore: ye are of more value than many sparrows" (Luke 12:7).

"For thy sake we are killed all the day long; we are accounted as sheep for the slaughter. Nay, in all these things we are more than conquerors through him that loved us. For I am persuaded, that neither death, nor life, nor angels, nor things present, nor things to come, nor any creature shall be able to separate us from the love of God, which is in Christ Jesus our Lord" (Romans 8:36-39).

That paper gave me a sense of security in Him and helped me to be brave. I admit, I was scared.

After the surgeon checked me out on Monday, he gave us the choice of waiting to see what happens or to do surgery. We felt ready to have it taken care of, so we signed for surgery, as he felt it was an 80% chance of it being an ectopic. He guessed the reason I wasn't having more pain was because the pregnancy was at the very beginning of the tube and had relieved the pain by moving slightly out of the tube. That or it was somewhere outside the tube. He gave us hope of saving the tube.

It turned out, though, that he couldn't save the tube, as the pregnancy had grown fast to the finger-like projections at the beginning of the tube. He had to remove the tube completely because it bled too much when he removed the pregnancy. I came home Monday night.

It was very shocking to us and I felt the loss greatly. I couldn't stand to look at babies for days afterward and I was very weak and emotional.

The day following the surgery was a day of misery. My stomach was still swollen from the gas they used and it pushed up into my rib cage so hard that I had to stay completely relaxed and take only small breaths. At times I had to cry, which hurt so badly I could hardly catch my breath.

The next day was better, but I had severe gas pains. Gas-X helped some. But the pain medication from the doctor didn't help, so I quit taking it.

The following weeks were occupied with making cards in my sister-in-law's basement. It helped to get my mind on other things and it was a tonic to have someone to talk to. Days at home alone were hard and long for me.

I was strongly advised not to get pregnant for six months. But at five months I became pregnant! It seemed like a miracle to us!

As soon as I could, I did a pregnancy test, and when it showed positive, we went for blood tests three times in two weeks to make sure my levels are going up like they should. Also to make sure it's not an ectopic again. I am going on four months now and all seems well. I have morning sickness quite severely, while the other time there was none. What a blessing!

Why God Gives Grief

God gives to each of us some grief,
A sip from out its dregs.
But why He sends it? Oft the soul
This troubling question plagues.

Why can't our life be all of peace
And full unmeasured joy?
Why must the road be steep at times,
And thunderclaps annoy?

Aye! It's so when life evens out,
And rainbows shine again,
We'll understand the burdened look
And feel our brother's pain.

We'll know just what he's going through,
And help to lift his load,
And pray for him and walk beside
Him up the winding road.

For no one who has never felt
The stinging throb of grief,
Can ever to the anguished soul
Bring comfort and relief.

—*Denise Rhiems*

A TEAR FROM MY HEART